Praise for
Living Well with Chronic Illness

Even after decades of pastoral counseling, I found Deacon Cheu's book to be very enlightening. With chronic illnesses being so common among friends and parishioners, I realize that this book offers wisdom and sensitivity that might have been missing when I was younger. No matter what our age, it is never too late to become a more compassionate person and a better pastor. This interesting guide can help.

—Msgr. William Belford, Vicar of Clergy, Archdiocese of
   New York

Richard Cheu has written an invaluable book that helps guide people physically, mentally, emotionally, and spiritually through living with chronic illness, something many of us will face in our lifetime. He combines concrete steps you can take with examples of others who have faced chronic illness to give the reader a complete model for living. As someone involved for over 25 years in the health care industry, I highly recommend *Living Well with Chronic Illness*. It will benefit not only those who live with a chronic illness, but the caregivers and family members who love them as well.

—Scott LaRue, President & CEO, ArchCare

Living Well with Chronic Illness is written in a personal and reassuring voice, as it covers the many complex factors that follow a diagnosis of a life-altering or life-threatening illness. It offers vivid case examples and good suggestions for coping with enormously difficult circumstances. I appreciate especially Richard Cheu's attentiveness not just to patients' needs but also to the impact on the circle of caregivers. This book will help many.

—Rev. Paul A. Metzler, D.Min., Director, Community
  Education and Spiritual Care Coordinator, Visiting Nurse
  Service of New York, Hospice and Palliative Care

I am finding it beautifully written and very poignant, valuable information — and timely.

—Margaret Wakeley — Community Development
  Coordinator, Gratefullness.org.

Living Well with Chronic Illness

LIVING WELL

with

CHRONIC ILLNESS

A Practical & Spiritual Guide

RICHARD CHEU

Dog Ear Publishing

First published by Dog Ear Publishing
4010 W. 86th Street, Ste H
Indianapolis, IN 46268
www.dogearpublishing.net

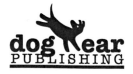

ISBN: 978-1-4575-1343-5

This book is printed on acid-free paper.

Printed in the United States of America

DEDICATION

For Janey, my wife and
best friend.

We don't beat the grim reaper by
living longer.
We beat the reaper by living well.

— Randy Pausch, "The Last Lecture: Really Achieving Your
Childhood Dreams"

CONTENTS

FOREWORD

I first met Richard Cheu years ago through a mutual friend, a psychologist. He introduced us to each other because Richard and I have both witnessed quite a bit of human suffering and share a passion to help those in need — he as a chaplain, caregiver, and patient advocate, and I through twenty-five years as a physician, chief of an acute psychiatric inpatient unit, a researcher focused on emotional traumas resulting from disasters, and producer of a documentary about earthquake survivors.

Richard immediately struck me as a man of immense humility and accomplishment. I found him to be deeply insightful in our many subsequent conversations about trauma, human suffering, resilience, and mortality. I consider Richard both a mentor and a friend and would like to believe that I have in some small way contributed to the blueprint for this book, especially since our divergent experiences have converged in our conversations.

There are countless ways that readers of *Living Well with Chronic Illness: A Practical & Spiritual Guide* will benefit from Richard's authorship and the guide itself. Richard has taken on one of the most important aspects of humanity that many of us refuse to face or hide from until it is too late. The concept of mortality and the fear of illness and death are ridden with complexity. We find them uncomfortable, so it is natural that we procrastinate and avoid embracing them.

Coming to terms with these concepts can enable us to live life—the here and now—to the fullest. Richard's guide provides the framework to do just that, and preferably, sooner rather than later. He provides instruction and tools to increase consciousness and see illness not as a barrier but as an opportunity. Real-life examples of those who have transformed themselves are contrasted with those who have not.

As a physician who practiced medicine and surgery in a third-world country prior to becoming a psychiatrist in the United States, I have had the opportunity to see firsthand the impact of chronic and terminal illnesses such as strokes, cancers, amputations, and so on, and the emotional aftermath that patients and their families are left with. Needless to say, human suffering is a universal experience, regardless of the quality of medical care. Medical technologies and advancements are abundant in the U.S. but can be scarce in other countries. On the other hand, there are countries where family, community, faith, and spirituality compensate for the lack of advanced medical care, leading to better outcomes. In my experience, patients in more advanced countries tend to depend on medical technologies and may overestimate their ability to heal, feeling disappointed and frustrated with the limitations of medical care, which in turn can lead to depression, hopelessness, and pessimism. Richard quite eloquently discusses these subtle emotional experiences, which he terms "emotional baggage," and skillfully describes a pathway to emotional wellness, freedom, and joie de vivre. Many will find his practical self-help worksheets very useful.

The scope of applicability of the guide's paradigm of grieving components—"SARA" or Shock, Anger, Resistance and Acceptance—is also compelling. Not only does this paradigm apply to illness as it presents itself, but it also stands to reason that reaching acceptance in its elevated form applies universally to physical as well as mental illness, not to mention to those without any perceived illness whatsoever. For example, at my Integrative Center for Wellness in New York, emotional well-being is closely tied to one's understanding of aging and the physical limitations that come as a result. Having worked with hundreds of patients on this basis, I can attest to the need for the body of work that Richard has put forth in this book.

As a mental health provider and a physician for more than two decades, I have also worked extensively with people suffering from mental illness. There is little distinction between chronic physical and mental illnesses: malignancies of the mind are as incapacitating as those of the body. The struggles, challenges, and coping skills required are the same, so this book will resonate with patients, practitioners, and all levels of providers, family, and friends across the entire wellness spectrum.

Likewise, through my own experience of providing care to Pakistani earthquake survivors over a five-year period, I have witnessed the fallout of massive human suffering and physical and emotional loss, and observed the role of faith, religion, and spirituality in resilience as well as the importance of family, friends, and community in healing. The application of coping mechanisms and the grieving process are universal.

Each of us, no matter where we live in the world, no matter what our culture, will experience shock, anger, resistance and inevitably acceptance, as Richard describes.

As director and producer of the film documentary *The Wrath of God: A Faith-Based Survival Paradigm*, a study of survivors of the 2005 earthquake in Kashmir and Pakistan, I find many analogies between the survivors I interviewed and the chronically ill patients that Richard describes—especially how they bravely face devastation, loss, death, and physical limitation, and over time emerge from suffering and achieve some level of wellness and resilience.

One personal example that comes to mind of the individual's ability to transcend suffering and achieve wellness is that of my uncle, Bob Mamu, who died recently. He had been told more than thirty years ago that heart disease required him to drastically change his active life. He opted to accept the new limitations and moved from Lahore, Pakistan, to a village for a less stressful lifestyle. He spent the next three decades helping others—bringing education, healthcare, and technical training to women and the poor. At the end of his life, he had achieved an unprecedented level of accomplishment and was happy and at peace. I am sure all of us know similar people.

In our increasingly detached culture of media, entertainment, and relentless consumerism, we lack so many aspects of community and caring that have been the mainstays of the past. This book helps bring us back to those basic values and groundedness to face illness and achieve mental wellness. Captivating from the beginning, the guide is moving, emotional, and real. It is about coping and transformation, as well as the planning and structural approach required to achieve harmony and prepare oneself for the inevitable. Individual autonomy is given equal importance to the need for collectiveness, and the fine balance of both is clearly defined as part of the process of becoming mentally well.

We tend to underestimate how optimism can breed resilience and wellness. Richard's use of positive psychology to achieve living well is the right approach for anyone facing chronic illness. With limited time to delve deeply into entire histories, a short-term approach that applies optimism and introspection to move through trauma and decrease suffering is critical.

Lastly and worth repeating, this book addresses the psychological challenges of patients suffering from chronic illness but is not limited to them alone. Family, friends, colleagues and many others will benefit by facing the unpredictable, preparing for the future, and seizing the day, starting today.

—Samoon Ahmad, M.D.
Clinical Associate Professor, Department of Psychiatry, NYU School of Medicine; Founder, Integrative Center for Wellness, New York

ACKNOWLEDGMENTS

I would like to express my grateful appreciation to the following people: Rev. Philip Marani, O.Carm., and Rev. Frederick Otieno Nyanguf, AJ, my hospital chaplain mentors who taught me to see the world through the eyes of the patient; all the patients and their families who allowed me to journey with them; and Peter Micheels, author and psychologist, for his many pearls of wisdom.

Part 1

THE PERSONAL IMPACT OF A

CHRONIC ILLNESS

CHAPTER 1

Answering Yes to Life: Expand Your Vision Beyond Your Illness

EACH TIME I WALK THROUGH the emergency department—something I do several times each day on my rounds as a hospital chaplain—the scene is different and constantly changing. There is a unique rhythm and tempo in each of the different ERs—pediatric, adult, fast-track, psychiatric, trauma—that creates an unfolding drama played out by a changing cast of patients and medical staff. At any given moment, there may be as many as a hundred patients being treated in the emergency department, another twenty-five people waiting in the walk-in reception area, and a half dozen who have just arrived by ambulance. Add to that dozens of patients in the intensive care unit, and you have an impression of the intense activity of an often impersonal big-city hospital.

At the center of this flurry of activity is a human being caught up in a personal drama of large proportion, possibly life or death, but certainly critical. When the day is done — when the doctor has delivered the diagnosis and prognosis and some urgent decisions have been made — this human being will be left with an overwhelmingly complex array of emotions, information, challenges, problems, and more decisions to be made. No wonder then that for many people, the first reaction to receiving a diagnosis of a serious illness is shock, followed quickly by fear, grief, helplessness, and despair.

It is my job as a chaplain to help people through their powerful initial emotions so that they can begin to deal with the long series of decisions and practical problems that will soon follow. I work with people at all stages of illness, from those who have just found out that they have a serious illness; to those who have been floundering helplessly for months, trapped in negative emotions and unable to make any sense of what is happening to them; to those who are nearing death. At each of those stages, there is important emotional, practical, and spiritual work to be done.

My mission is not just to help people survive their initial shock, or to trick them into feeling good about a bad situation by offering them spiritual promises. My mission with the patients I have the good fortune to work with over time is to help them remove whatever is blocking their heart and mind, gather their resources, develop a vision for what is to come — whether they have one week, one year, or many years ahead of them — take action, and create meaning out of all that is happening to them. In a word, I help people be at peace with their illness and all the changes it brings into their lives. For me as a chaplain, "peace" and "spirituality" are almost synonymous.

Joan and Jack

As I make my daily hospital rounds, how do I know which patients want me to stop and visit with them? The patients tell me with their eyes. There is a saying that says, "The eyes are the mirror of the soul." I find, however, that the eyes are more like the colored lights on a traffic signal that say, "Go ahead and talk to me," "Approach me with caution," or "Stop—I don't want to talk to you." Sometimes it is a nurse nodding toward a patient she thinks I should visit. Prisoners handcuffed to their stretcher, on the other hand, are focused on a personal agenda that doesn't involve me, and they don't really see me even when they look at me as I walk by. Most often, what I see in the patient's eyes is fear or anxiety, mirrored by the behavior of the friend or family member at the patient's bedside.

So one day I was rather surprised to look in an examination room and see a very relaxed middle-aged couple pleasantly chatting together, seemingly oblivious to the ER activities swirling around their island of calm. I stuck my head into their room, smiled, and said, "Hi. Can I come in?" They answered, "Certainly."

Joan and Jack were from the Midwest and had planned their trip to New York for several years. They were looking forward to seeing all the sights, especially Times Square.

Shortly after their arrival, Joan developed a strong stomach pain that just wouldn't go away. Jack worried that she had food poisoning and insisted she go to a hospital to be checked out. Joan was admitted to the ER and examined, received some medicine for the pain, and underwent several tests. Joan and Jack were patiently waiting for the test results and were very happy to chat with me about their trip.

They were a very amiable couple and easy to talk to. They told me about their lives back home, their family, and how they chose to come to New York to celebrate their thirtieth anniversary. They ran a small retail business together that required a lot of day-to-day attention, and the years just flew by. Now that the children were grown and on their own, they decided that the time had arrived for that big holiday trip they had been dreaming about for so long.

Suddenly a doctor and an assistant walked briskly into the room. Their demeanor instantly changed the atmosphere. The doctor introduced herself to Joan and Jack, apparently not seeing me sitting directly in front of her, and then directed her comments to Joan. She explained the purpose of the tests, paused, and then said compassionately but briefly, "I'm sorry to tell you that the test results are positive. It appears that you have cancer that has spread throughout your abdomen. A doctor from the cancer team will be in shortly to talk to you about possible treatments." When she finished speaking, I introduced myself. She said, "I'm sorry I interrupted your conversation," and strode out of the room.

Joan and Jack didn't say a word. They just looked into each other's eyes as they clutched hands so tightly that the skin blanched. In the blink of an eye, we went from happy chattering to not speaking. There was a terrible silence. Even I was taken aback by the brutality of the doctor's news intruding upon this couple's happiness. It was as if the doctor had turned off the light in the room. As Joan and Jack held each other, they "pulled up the drawbridge" and withdrew into themselves, leaving me the stranger on the outside of their lives. They asked me to pray with them and then I left as their tears began to flow. I knew they needed to be alone with their grief for a time.

When I visited Joan and Jack again later in the day, they were very different from the lighthearted vacationers I first met. Now the conversation was about more testing and treatment options. We did not talk about what was clearly hovering in the room: the specter of death. Joan was acutely aware of her body and her pain. She wanted to be released as soon as possible to fly home to family and friends. By the next day the anniversary couple had left New York City as quickly as they had arrived, returning to a familiar environment from which they could draw strength to deal with the realities of Joan's illness.

Suddenly, Nothing Is the Same

We can all remember where we were and what we were doing at important moments in our lives. Our minds are like camcorders that record our experiences in high definition, available for instant replay. You can probably relive the moment when the doctor told you that you have a serious illness that cannot be cured and vividly remember your reaction to that diagnosis.

You understand how Jack and Joan felt at that abrupt turning point in their lives. First the terrible news that unleashed a storm of emotions. Then the struggle to control their emotions while taking the first urgent steps to reorganize their lives to cope with unending change—changes no longer governed by their retirement plans, but by the progress of Joan's disease. To Jack and Joan, and perhaps to you, it felt as if they were riding in a wagon drawn by a team of panicked horses running full speed and senselessly along a dark trail. They felt that they had no control over their lives, a deep feeling of helplessness.

A major long-term illness changes everything, suddenly, in one fell swoop. It wipes clean many of your prior plans, hopes, dreams, beliefs, expectations, and daily routine. It changes who you've always thought yourself to be. Your secure base of everything you counted on and assumed would endure for some time is pulled out from under your feet. Suddenly you must completely change your focus, along with your priorities. It no longer matters whether the front porch gets painted this summer, or the lawn is mowed, or your socks match. Your attention is completely taken up by urgent medical and financial matters: doctors' appointments, x-rays, treatment plans, medications, baffling insurance paperwork. The list of things to do becomes endless, while you feel your energy diminishing.

Meanwhile, you are submerged in a pool of dark emotions: helplessness, fear, anger, stress, anxiety, grief, depression, loneliness. You have an acute and unwelcome awareness of your vulnerability and mortality. But there is barely a moment to attend to any of those feelings as you are overwhelmed by the practical demands of your illness.

It is no wonder that Joan and Jack held onto each other for dear life when Joan received the news that she had a cancer that would most likely be terminal. Faced with undeniable odds against our immortality, we instinctively do what our ancestors did thousands of years ago: we draw together for protection against a hostile universe.

The Antidote to Helplessness: Coping and Transformation

I have written this book for every person who is struggling with a severe or chronic illness at any stage, be it long-term or terminal. This book is equally for the families, friends, colleagues, doctors, and caregivers of people with serious illnesses.

This is a book about *coping* and *transformation*. The antidote to feelings of helplessness and despair is to come to terms emotionally with what is happening to you, adapt to the inevitable changes you will undergo, take action to have the best possible outcome, and find new meanings in your changed situation. Illness (like life) is about change. Coping is about successfully adapting to change. You work with the changes brought on by illness in order to have maximum control over the outcome — over your fate and your state of mind and heart. This process involves personal transformation on an emotional and spiritual level.

The mind and body immediately react to a devastating diagnosis by eliciting two powerful and ancient survival mechanisms: the fight-or-flight response and the grieving reaction. If allowed to continued for very long, these responses will severely handicap your ability to cope with your illness. The first step in coping is to bring the survival responses under control. Only then can the rest of the coping and transformation process successfully proceed.

I would like you to know at the outset that I fully understand your feelings of grief, depression, fear, and hopelessness. I have witnessed them in hundreds of people with severe medical problems and I understand how it feels to be trapped in feelings of despair and impotence.

My goal is to help you see that the "wild horses" of a chronic illness can be reined in. I will show you how to deal with the strong emotions generated by your illness; open your mind and heart to personal change; create new meaning from and for your past, present, and future; and use spirituality as a resource if you so choose.

Coping is the sum of all the things you do each and every day to live your life as best as you can in the face of all the constraints and burdens of your illness. Life with a chronic illness is very complicated and extraordinarily demanding of time and energy, a fact often not appreciated by people who have not had a personal encounter with a major illness. Unlike a treatable acute illness that has a defined course of treatment and predictable time frame, dealing with a chronic illness is like trying to solve a complex mathematical problem involving many different factors that must all be considered at the same time. The many and continuous burdens of your illness on you and your caregivers can be overwhelming. It is not unusual to hear patients say, "This illness is wearing me down" or "It's just too much for me to bear."

In my work with chronically ill patients, I have developed a practical and spiritual approach to help them take control of their illness and their life. It is based on my experience and training as a neurophysiologist who has taught medical and nursing students, an Emergency Medical Technician (EMT) with twelve years of street experience, an EMT instructor, and an ordained hospital chaplain serving at Bellevue Hospital, Mary Manning Walsh Home, and the Visiting Nurse Service of New York inpatient hospice.

In this book I will guide you through the stages of the coping process, from the initial shock you feel when you first receive your diagnosis, to overcoming the emotional hurdles that stand between you and your goals and aspirations, achieving a new perspective, setting new goals, and finding new meaning for your life. You will get to know some inspirational people who, like you, have dealt with a major illness and found ways to leave their mark on the world.

You may well find during this process that the illness you initially thought meant the end of everything that has been important to you turns out to be an opportunity for personal renewal that will lead you to focus more clearly on who you want to be and how you want to live your life.

How Many Suitcases Can You Carry?

You are now entering a new phase of your life. You are going to need every ounce of available energy and focus to confront your illness and all that it entails. The first key to successfully coping with a major medical problem is to let go of whatever is weighing you down and encumbering your mind and your heart. Imagine a person who has just spent many years working in Alaska and is transferred by his company to Hawaii. As he boards the plane with his suitcases, he logically leaves behind all the trappings of his life in Alaska that will not be needed in Hawaii — the snow boots, gloves, hats, snowshoes, skis, and so on. It would make no sense at all for him to drag those unneeded items into the next phase of his life, no matter how attached he may be to them.

Nor can you afford to carry around your excess emotional baggage as you take on this next stage of your life. The lighter your burden, the more energy and resources you will have for dealing with the important issues of your life. In reality, this is very hard to do when you are healthy. When you are sick, it becomes even harder because we tend to hold tight to what we know, even when it is hurting us, and are resistant to doing something new and different even if it will help us. The types of baggage I am talking about include fear, anger, unwillingness to acknowledge the changes in your life, inability to forgive, clinging to old animosities, unresolved grief — the list goes on and on. If your burden is heavy enough, it will simply stop you in your tracks: you will be immobilized and unable to cope with your illness. Together we will take a hard, honest look at your unnecessary mental and emotional burdens and get rid of as many of them as we can.

Once you've done that, you will be able to tap into internal strengths, wisdom, and resources that you probably don't even know are there, deep down inside you. And once you've stripped away thoughts and feelings that no longer serve you well, you will be free to live in the present and create new meaning for your life, a new way of understanding why you are here and how you want to carry on with your life.

Your Spirit Will Sustain You

This is a completely nondenominational book, but as a chaplain I can't leave out the role of spirituality in negotiating this phase of your life. I want to appeal to everyone who is searching for ways to take control of their life during a major illness, regardless of your religious beliefs. I have counseled hundreds of people of many faiths and of no faith. I have noted that there is one thing that we all have in common: we all long for peace of mind. We could spend days discussing the definition of spirituality and the best way to be spiritual, but a simple longing for peace of mind is what underlies all spirituality. If you don't want to call that "spirituality," then call it by whatever term resonates with you. Your body may be suffering, but your spirit is untouched by illness; it is there to sustain and uplift you. Please don't deny yourself the comfort of peace in your heart just because of someone else's terminology. Make your own spiritual language.

My objective is to help you to become spiritual; that is, to achieve a state of mind in which you are at peace with yourself, at any point of your life, and in spite of what your illness is doing to you physically. I invite you to embark on a journey to discover what it means to you to be alive in this world, the meaning of your illness, and the nature of your relationship to whatever is beyond you. It will be up to you to decide the terms of your search for peace and how you will live out your spirituality in this new phase of your existence. I will make suggestions for internal and external sacred places that can enhance your odyssey.

You can best undertake this journey with a free and open mind. That begins with letting go of whatever is weighing down your heart and mind. We will do that together, so that you may begin your journey toward taking control of your life and making new meanings for this new phase as unencumbered as possible.

Styles of Coping: You're in Charge

Grief counselors often say, "There is no right or wrong way to grieve." Everyone grieves in their own individual way. The same can be said of coping. You choose how you will cope with your illness. As a chaplain, I do my best to honor the differences in personality, spiritual beliefs, and life experience that lead the patients I work with to make very different decisions about how they handle their illness. And yet, it is also my role to help people thoughtfully decide how they will manage their lives, according to consciously chosen values and goals, rather than being led by negative emotions of fear, anger, and grief.

How you choose to respond to your illness goes beyond yourself and has a large impact on the people who form your support community. If it takes a village to raise a child, then it takes an army to support and care for a chronically ill person. The soldiers in this army — a mix of professional healthcare providers, volunteer caregivers, family, and friends — make a long-term commitment to service on your behalf, aware that there may be long periods of endless drudgery punctuated by unforeseen emergencies. All strive to adjust to your continuously changing world. Your family and friends may be deeply impacted by your illness, both emotionally and practically. Coping is therefore a balancing act in which you seek to address your own needs while maintaining an awareness of how your actions will impact those who are supporting and caring for you. In some instances, you may benefit more by taking actions for the sake of your support team than for yourself.

If you have a serious chronic illness, you already know about the complexity of all you must deal with now: your medical treatment, emotional and spiritual well-being, family matters, finances, interruptions to your career, and much more. No wonder the patients I counsel feel confused, overwhelmed, and often in despair! I believe I will be able to show you a way out of your confusion, if you will commit to approaching your illness with an open mind and entertaining new ways of thinking about yourself and your life.

My point is that although each person's situation is different, and therefore each person will choose a unique way of coping with their illness, for YOU there is a best way, a way that will best meet your individual medical, emotional, spiritual, and other needs; help you make sense of this very difficult time in your life; and bring you the serenity you seek. My purpose in this book is to help you find that way.

To illustrate my point, I would like to tell you the true stories of two seriously ill people who chose very different ways of handling their illnesses. Sadly, both passed away in the end, but because of the decisions they made in their final months the impact of their illness on themselves and their families, friends, and colleagues, and the legacy they left behind were very different.

I have changed the identity of the first person significantly to protect her family's privacy and out of compassion for her suffering. You may know the second individual—his story touched literally millions of people. As you read these true stories, I would like you to begin imagining how you will choose to respond to your illness from this moment on. How brave will you be in facing the reality of your medical prognosis and how you are changing? Will you shut out your loved ones, or be mindful of how much they need to be with you now? Will you try to create new meaning from your experience of illness, or will you close your mind against it? Will you be inspired or defeated by your illness? The choice is yours, as these stories will illustrate.

Sharon: Holding onto Life without Knowing Why

Sharon was a Type-A overachiever from the word go. When she graduated from high school she was designated "Most Likely to Succeed." She went to Columbia University on a full scholarship, graduated first in her class, and went on to do an MBA. At age twenty-five she was hired by a prominent Wall Street firm and placed on a fast track to an administrative position. For the next seven years Sharon defeated every challenge in her path, until she was promoted to assistant vice president.

Until that point, Sharon was driven by a single-minded devotion to her career. She worked eighty-hour weeks, six days a week. She did get married, but made a decision not to have children. It never occurred to her to ask whether she was living a full and complete life. She never inquired about the deeper meaning of the path she had chosen. It just seemed like the right thing to do, given her intelligence, her skills, and her drive.

When Sharon was thirty-two she received some news that she could never have imagined: she was diagnosed with breast cancer. She took little time to reflect on this news. She knew immediately what she had to do: push this obstacle out of the way and continue pursuing her life goals. She knew in her heart that she was strong enough to beat breast cancer. She felt unstoppable.

Sharon refused to talk to her doctors about the status or treatment of her cancer. She could not tolerate their pronouncements about how serious it was. Instead she delegated to her husband, Andrew, the responsibility of getting information about her cancer from her doctors and negotiating her treatment, using him as a physical and psychological buffer. She insisted that Andrew tell her only a bare minimum of details about her illness. She chose the most aggressive course of treatment.

Sharon's doctors noted that she did not cry when she received her diagnosis. She barely flinched during her treatments. She turned down all offers of psychological and spiritual care. In Sharon's mind, she was being strong. In truth, she was in denial. She could not, would not believe that her breast cancer was anything more than a slight blip on her radar screen. She may have been inwardly terrified, but she did not allow herself to feel or express those emotions. To Sharon, illness was a personal failure, and failure was not part of her mindset.

Sharon felt vindicated when her breast cancer was eradicated. She returned to her career with renewed vigor. At age forty-five she was finally promoted to CEO of her Wall Street firm, the youngest person and the only woman to ever hold that position.

Just two years later it was discovered that Sharon's cancer had spread throughout her body. This time she realized that she could not continue working. Her doctor recommended that she enter a hospice, but Sharon refused. Even though her doctors told her she had only months to live, she underwent a long series of painful treatments knowing that there was only a 1 percent chance that they would prolong her life beyond a few months. You see, Sharon had always been among the 1 percent, and she still believed she would outwit her cancer.

Sharon refused to allow her family, friends, and colleagues to see her as she lost weight and her hair fell out from the radiation treatments. "They will see me when I'm back to my old self," she said. Her parents and siblings were not allowed in her hospital room in her last days. They never had an opportunity to say good-bye to Sharon. She would not even allow Andrew to tell her what she meant to him and how he would miss her. She would cut him off when he tried to speak of those things. Andrew said his good-byes only after his wife died in his arms.

Sharon's story is about an unexamined life that turned into an unexamined death, trapping her in isolation and unspoken despair. Her decision to deny what was happening to her also denied her the opportunity to express her fears about her illness, to draw meaning from it, and to choose a meaningful way of spending her last months and negotiating her passage from this life. She spent her last weeks in acute physical and unexpressed emotional pain. Her family and friends were denied the expressions of love and caring that they desperately needed. So much unnecessary pain and emptiness!

Randy Pausch: Living Large on the Last Stage

You may have heard of Randy Pausch, a computer science professor at Carnegie Mellon University in Pittsburgh and expert in virtual reality and computer-generated entertainment. He is best known for a lecture he delivered in September 2007 entitled "The Last Lecture: Really Achieving

Your Childhood Dreams." He coauthored a best-selling book of the same title. His story was widely recounted in the news media because he wanted people to be inspired by how he chose to celebrate his life as he struggled with pancreatic cancer. He wanted people to take in the lessons of his own life.

Randy had some things in common with Sharon. Like her, he was a brilliant high achiever who found early success in his field. For students and colleagues alike, Randy was the model of a high-achieving young scientist destined for success and fame.

Randy was diagnosed with a very aggressive cancer in 2006 at age forty-six. In August 2007 his doctors told him he could expect just three to six more healthy months. From that point on, his decisions were the opposite of Sharon's in all ways. Rather than shutting his family out, he moved to another state to be closer to them. Initially, Randy rationally chose to try the treatments offered by his doctors. Unfortunately, the cancer quickly spread to other parts of his body. Rather than fight a battle that he would clearly lose, Randy stopped his treatment and died surrounded by his family on July 25, 2008. He was forty-seven years old. He left behind a wife and three children.

Soon after Randy learned that he had only three to six healthy months left, he prepared a speech called "The Last Lecture: Really Achieving Your Childhood Dreams," which he presented to a standing-room-only audience at Carnegie Mellon and also on the Oprah show. It was important to Randy to leave a legacy of life lessons and highlights of his life's work not just to students in his field, but to the world at large and especially his children. He wanted people to be involved in celebrating his life and in his final passage. He reached out as far as he possibly could to the world, and the worldwide response was enormous—his book entitled *The Last Lecture* has sold 4.5 million copies in the U.S. and was translated into forty-six languages; as of this writing the video of his lecture has been viewed more than eleven million times on YouTube! Accolades for Randy Pausch's "Last Lecture" and his major media appearances are simply too numerous to list. Suffice it to say that he inspired millions of people around the world with his dignified and impassioned path through his illness.

Randy Pausch's children, when they are older, will never have to wonder what he was like as a person, what was important to him, and how he lived out his final weeks. Randy took care to preserve a clear legacy for them, saying, "I'm attempting to put myself in a bottle that will one day wash up on the beach for my children."[1]

How to Beat the Grim Reaper

What Randy Pausch wanted to communicate was a love of life so strong that people would be inspired to pursue their dreams and persist through setbacks. While Sharon was focused on extending her life as long as possible no matter what the cost, it was without regard for the quality of that extra time, for her own understanding and solace, or for her loved ones. In his book Randy Pausch wrote, "We don't beat the grim reaper by living longer. We beat the reaper by living well." That message is true at all moments of our lives, even for those with a terminal illness.

The question is not whether Sharon's way of managing her illness was right or wrong according to my values. The question is whether her decisions brought her meaning, peace, and closer relationships. Sharon's decisions emanated from her inability to come to terms with her emotional pain. She adopted a blind course that shut her off from her own deepest needs when she most needed to be connected to them.

Randy Pausch took realistic stock of his situation, which allowed him to make deliberate, thoughtful decisions about how to manage his illness and how to spend his time. Although I want to offer my deepest compassion to Sharon, I think it is clear that Randy Pausch had the better outcome—for himself, his loved ones, and millions of people around the world.

I want to urge you to take a lesson from Sharon and Randy, two real people. Do not wall yourself off in solitude or a fixed mindset. Reach out to others in as many ways as you can think of. Examine your real needs and open your mind to all the ways the world offers you to meet them. Expand your vision as far beyond yourself and your illness as you can. Flow into this new life with grace and see where it takes you.

CHAPTER 2

Take Control of Shock, Stress, and Grief

IN THE FIRST DAYS AND weeks of living with your chronic illness, you will need to make many important decisions about your medical treatment, your finances, and more. To do that, you will need to have a clear mind. That can be difficult to achieve, especially in the beginning, because a chronic illness involves considerable stress and feelings of loss that can cloud your thinking. In this chapter we will look at how shock, stress, and grief manifest and what you can do about them.

A Devastating Diagnosis Is Like a Fire in Your Home

Have you ever witnessed the devastation caused to a home not only by the fire, but by the efforts of firefighters? I will never forget one fire I was called to during my years as a firefighter. A large hole had to be cut in the roof to vent the fire's superheated toxic gases. When I arrived, flames were shooting out of the second story and three hoses were spraying 375 gallons of water a minute on the extensive fire.

I entered the house hauling a hose with my team. We tramped across a fine carpet sodden with muddy water. As we climbed the stairs, a river of water cascaded down from the second floor. After we hosed down the flames, another team armed with poles tipped with steel hooks tore away areas of the ceiling and walls looking for hidden spots of fire. We did our job methodically and thoroughly. The fire was extinguished and we prevented it from spreading to nearby homes.

Afterward we descended the stairs to the first floor, passing by upholstered furniture saturated with the smell of smoke and a fine grand piano splattered with dirty water dripping through holes in the ceiling. Our chief congratulated us for our good work as we sat on the lawn recovering from our efforts.

It was then that I saw a man dressed in a silk bathrobe frantically running around the house, peering intently into the darkened interior. He held his hands to his head in despair and cried, "All my beautiful things are destroyed! Nothing will ever be the same!" Only then did I realize that this was the house of my music teacher. Until that moment I had not given any thought to who lived in that house and how they would feel upon discovering their ruined home. By necessity a firefighter's job is technical and impersonal.

If you have been diagnosed with a serious chronic illness, you can most likely identify with my music teacher's feelings of shock upon learning that everything he had built up over a lifetime had been wiped away by a fire. The news of your illness may have been completely unexpected, or you may have been noticing symptoms for some months and had a disquieting feeling about what was going on in your body. Whatever your circumstances, I have no doubt that this news was most unwelcome and that you had a strong emotional reaction to it.

As you saw in the introduction, medical centers are complex and very busy. Like firefighters, it is difficult for medical staffers to take a personal approach to each patient when they see hundreds every day. Their goal is to be technically competent in their work. Each staffer will know you only for a few moments as you are handed off from one testing or treatment station to another. You may feel you are just a number in a mass-production medical factory.

Regrettably, conditions in modern hospitals may greatly add to the stress and shock you feel when you receive your diagnosis. At the moment when you most need to see a familiar face and talk with a caring doctor who knows you well, you may feel alone and dehumanized. I strongly recommend that a friend or family member accompany you to your medical appointments.

The similarities to the fire I described may continue with your treatment. Like a fire, many illnesses can only be treated in invasive ways, so that the treatment may feel as bad as the illness itself. I don't mean to alarm you, but only to confirm what you have already experienced: that a serious chronic illness wreaks havoc in your life.

The Fight or Flight Response

When the doctor tells you, "I'm afraid I have some bad news," your world is turned upside down. In an instant you realize, like my music teacher, that everything has changed.

"Fight or flight" — a survival mechanism that developed in our ancient ancestors — is what is happening when you feel a rush of adrenaline, tension throughout your body, and rising emotions in response to a sudden stressor or shock. Your heart begins to race. Your breathing steps up. You begin to sweat. Your senses become more acute and you feel very alert. It is quite an unpleasant sensation.

This would all be very helpful if you were in the middle of the jungle and a lion were crouching twenty yards away. But we modern humans automatically go into the fight or flight state when we are not under immediate threat of dying, and this is not a good thing. Chronic stress causes the release of excess corticosteroids, which take a large toll on the body and mind in the form of irritability and anger, high-risk or compulsive behavior, sexual dysfunction, difficulty sleeping, depression, memory loss, and difficulty performing formerly routine activities. The most significant consequence is a weakening of the immune system. This is detrimental to anyone's health, but especially for the chronically ill patient.

For a chronically ill patient, the initial shock of the diagnosis is followed by a constant stream of trips to the hospital for tests and treatment. The body may remain in a continually elevated state of tension known as chronic stress. The human body has a unique capability to heal itself under moderate physical and mental conditions, including moderate stress. Sustained high levels of stress, however, can be damaging and even life threatening.

What to Do about Your Fight or Flight Stress Response

Since you are likely to face frequent stress related to your illness, it's important to develop stress-management strategies early on. You won't be able to make good decisions about your care and your life until you are calm and can think clearly.

When you're having an extreme stress response, your body is sending distress signals that your mind is interpreting as an acute emergency. So the first step is to calm yourself physically. Below are two methods of immediate stress reduction. They are simple to use and very effective. Choose the method that best fits your situation.

1. Control your breathing. Hyperventilation is a fight or flight response and will only make your stress feel more acute. One of the most effective ways to calm your physical response to stress is to take slow, moderately deep breaths. Try this right now and notice that as few as three deep breaths will change how you feel both physically and emotionally.

2. Visualization. There are many situations related to your illness that you would just rather avoid, aren't there? Some of those literally "get your blood pressure up." Some people have a rapid negative response, especially an increase in blood pressure, to exposure to medical settings and personnel. This is referred to as White Coat Syndrome.

Visualization takes you away from a stressful situation for a short time by putting you in a state of deep relaxation. It is a very simple technique. If, for example, you hate having your blood drawn, close your eyes, take several deep breaths, and imagine yourself in a relaxing and pleasant environment. See, feel, and hear everything as vividly as possible. Picture yourself sitting on a warm, sunny beach. Hear the waves rolling in and the seagulls. Feel the sun on your face, the sand under your feet. Allow those pleasant feelings to wash over you. When the blood has been drawn, simply open your eyes and return from the beach to the examination room.

You can use visualization anytime you want to reduce your stress level and are not doing something that requires you to be alert and attentive, such as driving.

I was asked to help a man who wanted to join a health club. The club required new members to have a blood pressure test. This gentleman repeatedly experienced White Coat Syndrome when his blood pressure was taken and he was rejected by the club. After a ten-minute lesson on visualization, he returned to the health club and successfully passed his blood pressure test.

Learning visualization also helped a church choir member, who was a very experienced singer with a beautiful alto voice, overcome her terror of performing solo. I taught her a visualization method that she used daily prior to the next church service. That Sunday she sang her solo effortlessly. Afterward she told me, "It wasn't stressful at all. I really enjoyed it and I'm going to do it again."

It's important to remember that fight or flight is an exaggerated response that goes well beyond the actual threat of the situation. Think of it as a false 911 call. Remind yourself to quiet the physical stress signals and then think the situation through calmly.

What to Do about Long-term Stress

In addition to the above strategies for controlling feelings of panic, it's important to build relaxation into your daily life. Identify the activities that give you a feeling of peacefulness and do at least one each day. Some suggestions:

- Meditation
- Walking
- Listening to or playing music
- Reading
- Spending time with family and friends
- A craft or other hobby
- Writing in a journal
- Pets

The methods described here are simple fixes for simple situations. If you find yourself experiencing prolonged and elevated stress levels that you are unable to bring under control, you should seek professional counseling.

The Grief Reaction

Grief is another response to a devastating situation that is automatic and universal. While you may think of grieving as undesirable, perhaps unbearable, it is actually necessary and positive. Like stress, grief is accompanied by strong biological reactions that can damage mental and physical health over time. The grieving process allows those biological reactions to subside over time.

The experience of veterans of warfare shows why grieving is necessary, and what happens when it is delayed too long. Soldiers in the midst of combat cannot afford to take time to grieve, because that would reduce their effectiveness and increase their chances of being killed. Grieving must be delayed until the soldier is no longer involved in combat. But at that point the feelings of grief are deeply embedded and may be experienced as too painful to talk about. Many people can tell the story of a relative who returned from war and refused to talk about his combat experiences or to discuss his grief over comrades who died in battle.

Sixty-five years after the event, an eighty-three-year-old veteran of World War II described landing at Omaha Beach in Normandy on D-Day. "The enemy gunfire was so intense that guys were being killed on our boat as we approached the beach. Officers, noncoms, medics—everyone was being killed left and right as we tried to move up the beach. There was total confusion. It was everyone for himself. It was horrible. I lost my best friends soon after we landed. I don't know how or why I made it and they didn't. I don't want to talk about it anymore."

Stages of Grieving

If you have been diagnosed with a chronic illness, you can most likely identify with the stress, shock and grief of that soldier, who was still haunted by unresolved grief sixty-five years later. He never had the opportunity to fully discuss what had happened and how he felt about it, so it remained with him all those years.

We now have a much better understanding of the components of the grieving process and can help people resolve their grief. In my work I use a paradigm called S.A.R.A. to help patients understand their grieving process when they are diagnosed with a chronic illness. The stages of grieving under the S.A.R.A. model are:

1. **SHOCK**
   "I can't believe it."
   "It's not possible."

2. **ANGER**
   "Why me? I live a healthy life."
   "Life isn't fair!"

3. **RESISTANCE** (DENIAL)
   "The doctors are wrong. I can beat this disease."
   "I don't want to talk about it."
   "There has to be a cure somewhere."

4. **ACCEPTANCE**
   "This is what I have to live with, so I will just make the best of it."
   "I'm taking life one day at a time."
   "Here's how I'm going to live my life."

Your Goal: The Acceptance Stage

The above stages, especially the first three, are very difficult for both the patient and caregivers. Shock, anger, and resistance can interfere with your doctors' efforts to treat your illness and with your family's efforts to care for you. The grieving process will help you heal emotionally so you can come to terms with your illness as soon as possible.

The purpose of the grieving process is to lessen your pain over time. Although we instinctively resist pain, you need to pass through the painful stages of Shock, Anger, and Resistance in order to arrive at the more peaceful stage of Acceptance. Your grief may never subside completely if your chronic illness has caused large losses, but if you will allow the process to take its course, your grief will gradually feel less intense and you will be able to function. You may even find that there is space in your life for happiness again.

The human heart has a natural healing mechanism. Over time new things come to take the place of what has been lost and we are able to feel happiness again. If you need proof that it is possible to accept a terrible illness, watch Randy Pausch's "Last Lecture" on YouTube. You will see that he experienced joy even in his last months of life. One reason for that is that he deliberately moved through the stages of grief and seized the time that he had left. He valued his remaining time and the quality of that time more than he valued his grief.

What Happens When We Don't Grieve?

If you resist your grief because you fear you won't be able to bear it, you can get stuck in the first phases of Shock, Anger, and Resistance and you will feel those unpleasant feelings over and over, in an endless circle. Imagine yourself walking round and round in soft soil. First a rut is created. Then a ditch. Each time a circle is completed, you sink a little deeper, until finally you are below the surface and can no longer see your surroundings. If you allow this to happen, you will end up in permanent grief that may cause depression and hopelessness, and a distorted perspective on your life.

Don't let your grief take control of your feelings, thoughts, and actions. Acknowledge your grief, but then gently nudge it out of the way and reclaim your life.

What Do We Grieve For?

As a person with a chronic illness, your grieving process is different from other forms of grieving. Usually we grieve for losses outside ourselves — a spouse, a pet, a home, a job. We can overcome those losses, remain intact, and continue on with our lives. But you are grieving for the most important person in your life: yourself.

When you are diagnosed with an illness that greatly changes your life, your first thoughts may be of all your dreams and anticipated experiences that may never happen. For older people, those may be all the wonderful plans they made for their retirement, after a lifetime of hard work. You think about all the important family milestones you will miss:

"I won't get to see my daughter walk down the aisle at her wedding."

"I won't see our son graduate from college."

"I'll never hold a grandchild in my arms."

You grieve for the person you were but are no more:

"I was such a good dancer then, and now I have to use a walker to get around."

"I was a well-known artist, you know. Now I can't hold a paint brush steady any more."

"I gave lectures without using notes. Now I have a hard time remembering things."

"I used to work seven days a week and never ran out of energy. Now it's hard to walk up the stairs to the second floor without tiring."

You grieve for lost opportunities:

"If only I had accepted the job offer, we could have been living the good life."

"We always wanted to travel in a mobile home when I retired. But I put off retirement to put more money in the bank. Now, we can't travel because of my illness."

Finally, you grieve because you are forced to face the fact of your mortality. Our instinct for self-preservation keeps our mortality out of our field of awareness most of the time. For many people, the sudden awareness of mortality when they fall ill comes as a shock.

Choose the Style of Grieving that Works for You

I would like to share with you two stories of people I have worked with to illustrate two different responses to grief — one that didn't work very well for the person, and one that did.

Frank had Parkinson's Disease and lived in an assisted-living facility. He developed quite a reputation as a still-life painter before his illness struck. He had a very pleasant personality and was easy to speak to. In our conversations, he told me how he developed his painting style and even gave me a signed print of one of his paintings. He had a very devoted family that visited him regularly.

As Fred's illness progressed, it became harder for him to paint the fine details in his still lifes. Upon my fourth visit with him he surprised me by saying, "I want to die." I was surprised because although Frank's illness had robbed him of the hand control he needed for fine painting, it was not progressing rapidly and his prognosis was not too grim. Naturally my first question to him was, "Why do you want to die?" He answered, "I can't paint anymore and painting is my entire life. Since I can't paint, I want to die."

Frank's situation was not unusual among the patients I work with. He had attained a level of success that he found personally and financially gratifying. He proudly wore a label identifying himself as an artist. When that label began to fade, he believed that there was nothing more for him in life. He was not able to tap into any other aspects of his identity. He couldn't see that he had other talents and skills that he could use now, even though everyone who met Frank saw his qualities, as did I. He reminded me of a diamond with only one polished facet, with others waiting to be cut to make the gem sparkle.

When I knew Frank, he was stuck in the second phase of S.A.R.A., Anger. He dug his heels in like a stubborn mule and could not be budged from thinking his life was over. His perspective did not waiver over the course of our meetings, and he remained frozen in his grief. He seemed to lose more of his spirit each time I saw him. This was a loss for Frank and everyone around him, as he still had so much to give and experience.

Louise's story was similar to Frank's but had quite a different outcome. Louise was one of the most interesting people I've worked with, but not the easiest. When I first met her she was mad — really mad! She had been a well-known pianist who had performed in the leading concert halls of the world. Her acquaintances populated the world of the rich and famous. She gave elaborate dinner parties at her beautifully decorated Manhattan apartment. Now she was forced to give up her glamorous lifestyle and live in a nursing home because of her debilitating C.O.P.D.

My first conversation with Louise was like standing in front of the open door of a blast furnace. Her anger was red hot.

"I can't stand this place! The food is terrible. Prisoners get better food than this. The walls of this room are closing in on me. There's nothing for me to do. I'm surrounded by boring people who haven't done a single interesting thing in their life."

"How do you know there aren't any interesting people here?" I asked. "Have you gotten to know any of them?"

"No, I haven't spoken to anyone. I can tell they're boring just by looking at them in the dining room."

"There are a lot of things to do here," I replied. "Do you think you would like to participate in any of the activities?"

Louise shot back, "No! I don't belong here!"

Our meetings went like that for many weeks as I listened to Louise vent her anger over and over. I invited her to explore her grief over losing her musical career with me, but she would immediately shut down the conversation. It was just too painful for her to talk about.

One day I arrived at the usual time and found Louise's room empty. When I inquired at the nursing station, I was told that she was at a writing class, which surprised me. The following week the nurse told me she was at her book club, and then a current events discussion group the week after that. This could not possibly be the Louise I knew. I was very curious to know what had convinced her to leave her room and take up these activities, but each time I passed by her room on my weekly rounds, it was empty.

About a month later, I happened to meet Louise coming out of an elevator. She looked greatly changed, almost radiant. We sat in the parlor and talked about what had changed in her life. She explained that one day she was sitting in her room, fuming as usual, when the thought came to her, "I can stay mad for the rest of my life or do something about this terrible situation. So I began by talking to a couple of people at dinner. To my great surprise, they had very interesting backgrounds and were good conversationalists. I was so surprised to discover that there are a number of interesting personalities in this place. One of them convinced me to try a writing class. I had never written anything in my life, but I love it!"

The real turning point came when a new friend led Louise to the grand piano in the visitor reception room and asked her to play something. "I played a couple of show tunes and before I knew it, there was a crowd around the piano and people were asking me to play their favorite song. Now I play for a few minutes every day before dinner. Everyone loves it and I'm having a grand time. Oh — and the food has gotten better."

If You Can't Play for Thousands, Who CAN You Play For?

Anger and Resistance are like quicksand: if you move through them too slowly, they can trap you permanently. I don't know if Frank ever moved beyond his anger and found new kinds of happiness. I know that Louise was able, over a period of months, to let go of her grief over the loss of her music career and find a new way of sharing her joy of music with people. She was no longer playing for thousands, but her music lit up the nursing home.

Louise certainly still missed her old life, but she found new joy in telling stories about the places where she had played and the people she had met. She began recording her stories in her writing class and eventually she turned those memories into a self-published book.

Louise was able to acknowledge that her life had changed and that it would never be the same again. She asked herself, "Well, if I can't play for thousands in London, what CAN I do?"

Louise's story shows that you can create new meanings from the things that have been important to you. Those things are never entirely lost. Later in this book I will show you how to make new meanings from your past and share them with others.

Part 2

OVERCOME EMOTIONAL HURDLES

CHAPTER 3

Life Is Change
(And Change Is Good)

The truth is that our finest moments are most likely to occur when we are feeling deeply uncomfortable, unhappy, or unfulfilled. For it is only in such moments, propelled by our discomfort, that we are likely to step out of our ruts and start searching for different ways or truer answers.

—M. Scott Peck, *The Road Less Traveled and Beyond: Spiritual Growth in an Age of Anxiety*

Change Is an Essential Part of Living

IN THIS CHAPTER I HOPE to persuade you that you can turn the changes brought on by your illness to your advantage by looking at yourself in new ways and welcoming change into your life.

You probably remember every detail of that moment when you realized that you have a chronic illness: where you

41

were, what you were doing, who was there with you, what was said or not said. You can recall that moment at anytime. This is true for everyone. The truly big events of our life are engraved in our memories in infinite detail, and the appearance of a chronic illness was a really big event for you. Chronic illness brought tremendous changes into your life that likely aroused some very strong emotions such as anger, fear, grief, and stress.

Sometimes it takes big changes in your life to hear and see the personal message attached to those changes. When changes in your life are small, it is easy to ignore them and pretend that they are not happening or, at the very least, not pay any attention to them. But when chronic illness entered into your life, you simply could not ignore its presence. It's like having a five-hundred-pound gorilla sitting in your kitchen: you may not like his presence, but he will continue to sit in your kitchen until you do something about him.

What if it turns out that this five-hundred-pound gorilla happens to be a gourmet chef who will take command of your kitchen and create wonderful meals to satisfy your every whim? No matter what you ask for, he knows how to prepare it and will even clean up the kitchen afterward. There is no entrée or dessert that he doesn't know how to prepare. Now that you know this, are you going to let him sit idle in your kitchen, simply taking up space, or are you going to put him to work to improve the quality of your life?

Chronic illness is very much like this gorilla: it can be a gigantic road block to living, or it can actually be an invitation to begin a new phase of your life that is more fulfilling and more gratifying than you can imagine at this moment.

To live is to change. Your body is continually changing, every moment of every day. Under normal circumstances, these changes are small and you are not aware of them. They don't interfere with your daily life or activities, so you come to believe that you aren't changing. But when you add up all these individual changes, they move you from one stage of life to another.

As you change physically, you also change how you interact with the world around you. Every time you come in contact with something in your environment — a television program, a magazine article, an e-mail from a friend, your various activities — your mind remembers each encounter as a picture in a mental photo album labeled "My View of the World."

Equally important are the times when you interact with yourself: when you are looking into yourself and thinking about some aspect of your personality or something you did or didn't do. Each of these personal encounters is recorded as a kind of brain picture in another mental photo album labeled "My View of Myself."

At some point in your life, you may begin to think about some important questions that are serious in nature and difficult for anyone to answer: What is the purpose of my life? Will it matter that I walked on this earth? To help you answer these and other equally important questions, your mind will sort through and select certain mental pictures to be placed in an album called "My Spiritual Self."

Why, you ask, do I have so many photos in each album? Wouldn't just one be sufficient? Before I can even respond, you already know the answer: <u>You are continually changing</u>

both physically and mentally. So every encounter with your surroundings or yourself is an entirely new event.

These mental photo albums are your personal property. You don't have to share them with anyone else, unless you want to. They are very valuable to you because you can use them to improve your quality of life and make yourself a better person in any way you wish.

Some people think that who and what they are is set for life, engraved in stone. That is simply not true. You can become anything you want to become and achieve anything you want to achieve, if you are willing to discard some of the images in your albums and replace them with new ones. You are in control of how you change or don't change. You are in charge of your future. Understanding that your future is under your control is very important to shaping how you respond to your illness.

The Benefits of Change

Patients with a chronic illness are susceptible to viewing the future as less positive than their past, especially after receiving their diagnosis. As we have discussed, this initial reaction is common and very much expected. However, if you have the desire to move beyond your diagnosis and pick yourself up mentally and physically, you will find yourself better off in several very important ways.

First, many people are initially shaken up by their diagnosis of a major illness, but you have probably heard many stories about people who used their diagnosis to transform themselves and their lives. Our language is full of metaphors that express these possibilities: "Turn lemons into lemonade." "Every cloud has a silver lining."

Is it possible that you were not living a full, purposeful life prior to your diagnosis? Your illness may turn out to be the motivation you needed to reevaluate what you want out of life, and what you want to give to life. Your illness will challenge you in many ways to help you become more aware of how you are living, handle problems and your emotions better, relate more positively and compassionately to the people around you, use your time more wisely, deepen your spiritual experience, and so on. Over time you will come to realize that you have changed for the better, that you are a richer and wiser person. This personal transformation may well open up new opportunities for you that you can't imagine at the moment.

Reread the quote from M. Scott Peck at the beginning of this chapter and see if you can find ways to apply it to your own situation. What ruts do you need to step out of? What new ways of living would serve you better? What answers are you still searching for? Use your illness as a catalyst for thinking about yourself and your life in new ways.

Second, you can definitely improve your quality of life by paying more attention to every aspect of how you are living and attending to your symptoms so that you can focus on a lifestyle that allows you to achieve your present and future goals. Like so many people, you may have been able in the past to live a carefree lifestyle without any thought of the consequences. The onset of chronic illness changed all that. Now you have to pay attention to the small details of living to take the best possible care of yourself.

Third, your willingness to adapt to changes in lifestyle for the sake of a better quality of life will yield a totally unexpected benefit: greater self-esteem. Every time you overcome your ever-present natural resistance to change and push forward with yet another small change, you score a point for yourself against your illness. I can tell you from personal experience that how you progress is just like climbing a mountain. Each time you move a foot up to a new foothold or a hand to a higher handhold and move up the face of a steep mountain just a few inches, this is a significant personal victory. Each small achievement motivates you to keep moving — one small victory at a time until you reach the summit. With each achievement, your self-esteem increases.

Greater quality of life and increased self-esteem are wonderful goals for everyone whether afflicted with a chronic illness or not. For you, however, there is an even more important motive for responding to change in very positive ways. How you respond to the changes brought about by your illness will determine your physical and mental health. A healthy body and mind are essential qualities for resisting and fighting back against illness. In other words, how you respond to change affects your illness. It's that simple, and you can do it: you can adapt to the changes in your life to have the best possible outcome to your illness.

Our Natural Reaction to Change

Your instinctive reaction to change is the result of many different influences interacting on you. Some of the most important influences are age, personality, family and social culture, past experiences, and people you know (coworkers, friends, acquaintances). Your response to change is uniquely and individually yours.

Psychologists have found that people tend to belong to one of five groups based on their adaptability to change:

1. Very Easily Adapt to Change
2. Easily Adapt to Change
3. Adapt with Ambivalence (They are not sure if they will benefit from adapting to a specific change.)
4. Adapt with Difficulty
5. Adapt with Great Difficulty

Interestingly, people move between these groups during their lifetime as their adaptability changes. They are most likely to change from one group to another because of the influence of two factors: age or life experiences.

The Influence of Age

Age is a very important factor in determining how we respond to change—especially with respect to self-esteem—at each stage of life, from infancy to seniority. These stages are a reflection of how our bodies are changing. From infancy through young adulthood, our bodies are growing with increasing strength and capabilities. It is in these early stages that we are most open to change, to taking a chance with something new that we have not yet experienced. It is no surprise that ski jumpers are very young. Adolescents and young adults are the most adaptable to change and accepting of the high risks associated with ski jumping.

In the stages of early adulthood, middle age, and seniority, people tend to become more conservative and less open to change. So they will move down to a lower category of change adaptability. Some of the growing reticence to change is the result of having less energy, body parts that don't work as well because of diseases associated with aging such as arthritis, and less strength with each passing decade. It takes work to stay physically fit as you grow older, and some people resist this effort.

The Influence of Life Experiences

Life experiences can shift your adaptability to change either upward or downward, depending on whether you think your previous efforts to adapt to change were successful or unsuccessful. It is the more significant events in your life that will cause this shift — a new personal relationship, marriage, the birth of a child, a new job, moving your residence, divorce, the death of a loved one or friend, job loss, retirement, or severe injury or disease. A successful life experience will increase your receptiveness to change and move you upward on the adaptability scale. An unsuccessful life experience will have the opposite effect and possibly bring about a negative emotional reaction — fear.

The Influence of Fear

Fear can be the greatest hurdle to adapting to the changes brought on by chronic illness: fear of the unknown, of suffering, of death, of being alone, and so on. Uncontrolled fear results in a fight-or-flight response and a heightened level of stress. Prolonged exposure to high levels of stress can weaken the body's defenses against diseases like cancer, heart attacks, and strokes. Try to keep in mind President Franklin Roosevelt's reminder to the American people in his first presidential inaugural address, at the height of the Great Depression: "The only thing we have to fear is fear itself." We will take an in-depth look at how you can work with and around your fear in chapter 4.

Change Can Be Good for Your Health

Are you among the many people who fantasize about winning the lottery? Do you buy lottery tickets even though your chances of winning are less than one in a million? That tells me that like most people you value wealth, and you think that acquiring great wealth is a matter of chance. Many people don't understand what wealth really is, nor how to accumulate it. Here are two basic principles of wealth that can greatly help you adapt to your chronic illness:

Wealth Principle #1: **Health is wealth.** Wealth can be defined as "what is most valuable and most important to you." Everything that is important in life depends on having the health to experience and enjoy it: your work, your relationships, your leisure activities, your independence, your finances. Without health those basic elements of your life are very limited or meaningless. For a person with a chronic illness, health is wealth!

Wealth Principle #2: **You decide how much "health wealth" to accumulate.** Unlike the lottery ticket holder, how much real wealth you acquire is not a matter of chance. You are not dependent on wishing, hoping, or the right combination of numbers inside a fortune cookie to acquire wealth. It is up to you to take steps to acquire that most important type of wealth called "health." You can decide when, how, and how much health to accumulate. Of course, this involves making changes in how you view yourself and learning exactly what health means for you.

If you really want to increase your level of health and quality of life, you will have to make changes in your lifestyle. You are most certainly aware that health depends on things like diet, exercise, reducing stress, and avoiding risky behaviors such as smoking and excess alcohol consumption. Perhaps you nod your head and agree that healthier habits would really be great, but you can't get motivated enough to make the changes necessary to acquire greater health. I am confident that once you realize the very significant benefits to be gained from changing your health habits, you will be motivated to do so.

The explorer Ponce de Leon is said to have been searching for the Fountain of Youth when he discovered Florida in 1521. Whether or not this story is true, it is certain that humankind has been seeking a way to slow or stop the aging process for thousands of years. In the twenty-first century, there are people who spend great sums of money on plastic surgery and

Botox injections to make themselves appear younger. Like those who buy lottery tickets, they are engaging in a fleeting fantasy. The regrettable difference is that there are no winners in the plastic surgery lottery. Aging processes occur internally, in the body and mind. The skin is merely one external reflection of those processes. You will need to look deeper, beneath the skin, to understand aging.

What Ponce de Leon didn't know was that it is possible to slow or even reverse the aging process by choosing specific behaviors that are within our control. Our behavior is the most accurate predictor of our biological age. A stereotypical description of a senior citizen might include: walks more slowly and has difficulty going up and down stairs; doesn't see very well, especially at night; is becoming deaf; retells the same stories from the past; is having a harder time remembering things and names; is out of touch with contemporary events and developments; thinking is slowing. This person is simply getting old, and plastic surgery will have no beneficial influence on any of these aging problems. However, adopting healthier life habits for body and mind can yield a fantastic benefit: slowing of the aging process. Here is a short list of lifestyle changes that can help you live longer and better:

- A program of regular exercise can improve muscle tone, strengthen your bones, and make walking easier and more enjoyable.
- Weight loss can reduce knee pain, making it easier to go up and down stairs. Losing just one pound reduces the pressure on the knees by four pounds.

- Getting the right amount of quality sleep can protect you from viral infections, heart disease, stroke, and mental decline.
- Eating right, exercise, reducing stress, and constantly challenging your mind can help you keep your mind sharp.
- A healthy diet strengthens the immune system, which protects against cancer.

That list could go on for several pages — there are literally dozens of things you can do to improve your chances of living longer, with greater quality of life.

In many cases lifestyle changes will have a direct positive impact on your chronic illness. Change can indeed be good for your health, so use your illness as a wake-up call to make these changes if they are overdue. Stop unhealthy habits now and substitute healthy daily habits, especially nutrition, exercise, sleep, and stress reduction.

Responding to the Changes Brought by Your Chronic Illness

Your chronic illness is likely to bring major changes into your life. The impact goes beyond bodily changes. You have undoubtedly noticed changes in your thinking, your emotions, and your spiritual outlook as well. You will find strategies for adapting to these mental, emotional, and spiritual changes throughout this book. Let's look now at practical ways you can adapt to your illness.

Understanding Your Disease

A chronic illness can leave you feeling that you lack control over your life and your own body. The first step to taking back control is to understand your disease. That will help you learn to manage it.

People usually speak about disease and illness as if they are the same. But they are not the same thing. A *disease* is a name (like "diabetes") given to a detailed description of a set of abnormal physical, chemical, and biological processes that are occurring in the body. Diabetes is a disease. These names are used by medical personnel as verbal shortcuts to communicate faster. If a doctor says to another doctor, "The patient has diabetes," the second doctor immediately understands what kind of medical problems the patient has. There are two kinds of diseases: those which can be cured (acute) and those which cannot be cured (chronic).

Illness refers to all the body's reactions to the disease that can be measured or are felt by the patient. We call these *symptoms*.

"My blood pressure is very high."

"I feel like the room is spinning."

"I have a hard time breathing."

Unchecked, your disease will continue to make claims on your health. If you want to compete with the disease for your body, you need to understand what the disease is doing now and might do in the future. When your doctors ask you for a decision about a treatment they are suggesting for you, it helps if you understand how the treatment might or might not help you.

Syms, a former chain of clothing stores in the Northeast, had a slogan that is very applicable for you: "An educated consumer is our best customer." There are many resources that can help you get the knowledge you need: frank discussions with your doctors, self-help medical books, the internet, and support groups where you can get information from people who have been successfully managing their illness — all will be helpful.

Managing Your Illness

The word "manage" sends chills down the backs of some people. I have a friend, Andy, who has been offered a promotion to manager many times. Each time he has refused the promotion.

"I like what I do," he says. "I'm very good at what I do. Managing other people is a messy business involving lots of changes and will take time away from what I really like to do." Andy is right, of course. Managing other people or yourself is "messy" because it involves responding to change.

If you think that managing the symptoms of your disease is beyond your capability, let me reassure you that you can do it once you've decided to <u>take control of the illness rather than letting the illness control you</u>. Perhaps the following story will help you believe in your abilities and inner strength.

Type 1 diabetes (formerly called juvenile diabetes) is one of the most difficult diseases for patients to live with. Managing the symptoms of Type 1 diabetes requires the patient to constantly monitor blood sugar level. This requires pricking the skin to draw a drop of blood to test the sugar level many times a day. Some patients, especially teenagers, prefer to deny that they have diabetes and do not keep their blood sugar under control. The results are uniformly bad and can even cause death.

I recently met with twenty-eight-year-old Phil Southerland in New York City to learn more about how he is inspiring Americans with Type 1 diabetes to manage their illness. He was diagnosed with diabetes before his first birthday. As a child, he was reckless and defiant about keeping his blood sugar under control. At age six, his mother made it abundantly clear (as only a mother can do) that if he continued to allow his blood sugar to fluctuate wildly, he would suffer great consequences and even death. Ever since, he has diligently controlled his blood sugar level.

Phil is an ardent bicycle racer. In college, he successfully convinced a fellow student racer with diabetes that controlling the blood sugar level would improve performance for a diabetic. In 2004 they decided to share this message with other young people by forming a professional racing team of diabetic cyclists. They called it Team Type 1.

The success of the team — over fifty first places in 2009, including the three-thousand-mile Race Across America — makes it easier to deliver a meaningful message to Type 1 diabetics, especially young people, who are naturally rebellious and resistant to the personal discipline required to keep their blood sugar under control. New teams have been formed, including a women's professional Team Type 1 and a Team Type 2.

Phil pointed out to me that diabetes is a very frustrating disease because of the need to constantly manage all the factors that affect blood sugar level. The message that he and Team Type 1 are delivering to all diabetics — "You can achieve your dreams when you control your blood sugar through diet and exercise" — is resonating with healthcare providers and diabetics of all ages.

Managing your illness is a team effort, somewhat like flying an airplane. As the pilot, you are responsible for setting a destination, preparing a flight plan, and controlling the aircraft to complete the flight safely. However, you can't do this all by yourself, even if you're flying solo. As an Air Force pilot once told me, "It takes ten people on the ground to keep one pilot in the air."

Managing your chronic illness is a lifelong flight that will include moments of frustration and flying through storm clouds. By working with the members of your healthcare team and persisting through the tough times, you can do it. How sweet the taste of victory will be when you can say that you ran the good race!

Change is difficult but necessary. If you feel resistant and resentful toward the unwanted changes that your illness has brought into your life, consider your resistance as an expectable — everyone feels this way — but only temporary stage. You will go through a series of phases as you come to terms with your illness. With each stage your understanding and your ability to cope will improve and you will figure out how to weave your illness into the fabric of your life. If you can open your mind to solutions and positive changes, you will be able to use your illness as a springboard for personal transformation on all levels. Your emotions, health, relationships, activities, and spiritual experience will all take on a deeper meaning that is closer to what you have really wanted for your life.

CHAPTER 4

Let Go of Your Excess Baggage

As you move from one stage of life to another, you cannot bring all your baggage.
— J. Wallace Sterling, *president of Stanford University,*
speaking at a student seminar in 1959

How Many Suitcases Do You Really Need for This Voyage?

IN THIS CHAPTER WE WILL examine the most common negative emotions—fear, despair, anger, shame and guilt, and loss of faith—and I will share with you specific ways for dealing with each one and how to let go of them.

The pearl of wisdom quoted above was offered to me many years ago when I was a student at Stanford University in a class called Historic Problem Solving, taught by our president. In one class meeting he discussed problem solving at different stages of life. I never forgot his comment about baggage, and it has served as the foundation of much of my pastoral counseling.

Almost everyone has experienced, at one time or another, the problem of having more things than we actually need for our immediate situation. When we travel we tend to bring along clothing that we never wear. We move to a new residence and have to throw out things that would not be of any use in our new home. Many people impulsively collect things that seem important at the moment and then stash them away, only to forget about them. Just look inside your closet or your desk and you'll know what I mean.

Wallace Sterling, however, was talking about a different kind of baggage. He was helping his students to focus on the *emotional baggage* that is created and attached to our every life experience, from the time we enter the world until the moment we leave it. Each experience is recorded in our memory as a mental photograph, painted with shades of different emotions that reflect how that experience impacted our life at that moment. Most images, even if painted with strong emotions initially, gradually fade with the passage of time. For example, an infant's strong emotional attachment to a baby blanket is an image a teenager prefers to forget. Your first love in high school is forgotten until someone mentions it at your twentieth high school reunion. You have thousands of these harmless memories.

Emotional baggage is the memory of an experience and the negative emotions attached to that experience. They are significant and worthy of your attention now, as you deal with your chronic illness, because they make it difficult for you to travel on your life journey. They slow you down, they are stressful, they waste your precious energy, and they harm your health — just like a huge suitcase full of unneeded items that you carry from city to city on a trip. In this chapter I will help you get rid of that extra suitcase to lighten your load as you move forward.

Why Excess Emotional Baggage Is So Harmful

Negative emotions are a problem for everyone, but they are especially burdensome for anyone with the added mental weight of dealing with a chronic illness. A list of common negative emotions could be as long as your arm. In this chapter we will focus on six specific ones that can be very difficult to deal with and very hard for some people to shed: *fear, despair, anger, shame and guilt,* and *loss of faith.*

Fear can stop you from moving, mentally and physically. It casts a shroud over your mind that causes mental blindness — an inability to see down the road — and prevents you from seeing opportunities for improving your quality of life. In the enveloping darkness of fear, the mind can become confused and doesn't know which path to follow.

Despair leads to a loss of hope which is the basis of life. When a person loses hope, death of the spirit and possibly even the body may follow.

Anger is very harmful to your health. It can arouse destructive thoughts of revenge aimed at specific people or organizations. It causes high levels of stress and anxiety. Anger damages your immune system and makes you vulnerable to very serious diseases such as cancer, heart attacks, and strokes.

Shame and guilt focus your attention on the past. If you are constantly looking backward, you can't expect to see the best path forward. In many instances, shame and guilt are the result of carrying someone else's baggage.

Loss of faith is particularly debilitating. It is the equivalent of losing your compass or map while traveling through unfamiliar territory. Faith, in its broadest sense, is simply what you believe in. Whatever you believe in provides the guidelines for how you live your life—including how you handle your illness. Without these guidelines, you lose sight of your goals and priorities and may engage in behavior that is detrimental to your health. Even worse, a loss of faith can lead to losing hope, which reveals itself in mental and emotional surrender to your illness: "I give up. I don't have the energy to fight this anymore."

Negative emotions are contagious—one quickly leads to another, and together they conspire to keep you in a negative state of mind. Fear can lead to anger or vice versa. Anger and fear together are a very powerful team that is hard to defeat. Add guilt to the mix and the combination is such a barrier to moving forward that professional counseling is often needed to defeat them.

Throughout this book I am encouraging you to use your illness as a cornerstone for personal transformation. Carrying around these types of emotional baggage is a real hindrance to that process, and I urge you to come to terms with them as early on as possible.

Why We Hold onto Our Excess Emotional Baggage

Fear is the Super Glue that binds negative emotions to your mind. It is such a powerful emotion that it can make you hold onto the past when there are much better options right in front of you. Perhaps you have experienced strong feelings of fear when you became entangled in the complexity and ambiguity of treating your illness: so many different possible treatments to sort through, their advantages, their risks and side effects, the likelihood of whether the treatment will be successful or not. At a time when you need the reassurance of certitude, your doctor cannot guarantee that the treatment will benefit you. It could even make matters worse.

As you try to decide whether to go ahead with the recommended treatment, you may be stymied by fear. For some people, fear of the unknown (the uncertainty of the treatment) is greater than fear of the known (the current condition of the illness). The fear of making a mistake can be so great that it shields your mind's eye from the potential benefits of the treatment.

There are many other reasons that may explain why you are holding onto excess emotional baggage: past unresolved traumatic experiences; personal, family, and cultural inhibitions; financial concerns; or simply not understanding what the doctor is telling you. Until you can successfully deal with the issues that are keeping you from moving forward, the associated negative emotions will remain a part of your emotional baggage.

The Benefits of Letting Go

Imagine you are engaged in a strenuous game of tug-of-war in which you are holding one end of a rope and all your negative emotions are gripping the other end. The rope is stretched across a ravine. When the game starts, you dig your heels into the ground and pull with all your might. But the negative emotions are too strong and despite your best efforts they are slowly but surely dragging you closer and closer to the brink of the ravine. If you fall in, you'll be trapped there forever! Suppose, however, that *you decide you don't want to play this game and you just let go of the rope.* Suddenly the weight is released as your opponent on the other side falls back. You are no longer threatened with falling into the ravine and you are free of the negative emotions.

There are a great many emotional, spiritual, and physical benefits to be gained if you are willing to sort through your baggage and toss out anything that may be blocking your health and peace of mind. A short list includes freedom from fear, gaining hope, calming the flames of anger, looking forward instead of backward, and gaining a sense of purpose that goes beyond your illness. You will be relieved to notice these changes in how you feel and in your ability to handle things:

- You will come out of the darkness of negative emotions into the light of day and see the world as it is.
- You will be more agile mentally because you have less to carry.
- Unburdened, you will have the capacity to add the positive baggage of new experiences.

- You will have greater self-esteem, which will help you deal with the past and plan confidently for the future.

Fear

Letting go of fear is one of the most powerful things you can do for yourself. When you let go of the fears that are connected with your chronic illness, you will toss away the heaviest pieces of excess baggage that you have been carrying and you will immediately receive enormous benefits from doing so. The first benefit is a sense of relief. You will ask yourself, "Why did I carry that tremendous and useless burden with me for so long? Why didn't I throw it away sooner?" The greater the fear, the greater the emotional release. Carrying that negative emotion is like trying to drive a car while pressing on the accelerator and the brake pedal at the same time. All this time, fear has been restricting your ability to move. Once you have rid yourself of your most oppressive fears, you will feel free. For some people, the sense of freedom is so great that it approaches a feeling of elation.

A second benefit of letting go of fear is your increased willingness to share what is really happening in your life with others. It is possible that you have hidden your fear behind a carefully created façade so that no one else can see it. But that means that no one can help you with the things that are troubling you. When you lower your façade and allow others to participate in your true feelings and the realities you are facing, you open yourself up to the emotional and practical support that you need. This support will make it easier for you to let go of whatever is blocking your forward progress.

A third and very important benefit of releasing your fears is the impact on your health. A heightened level of fear, which manifests both physically and emotionally, triggers a strong stress reaction. When that stress persists over a long period of time, it brings about physical changes that damage your body. It can cause high blood pressure, difficulty sleeping, irritability, loss of attention, vision problems, headaches, poor eating habits, and excessive alcohol consumption. Fear can also bring about depression that you can't shake, and you seem to spiral downward like an airplane out of control.

You can't afford to saddle yourself with any of those added physical burdens while you're trying to deal with a chronic illness. Letting go of fear will significantly improve your health immediately and over the long term and will increase your ability to deal with your illness.

A fourth benefit will be a growing sense of calm as you realize you have survived a threatening situation. As you work through your fears and release them, you will see the world in a more positive way. Opportunities that were not visible when you were cloaked in the darkness of fear will reveal themselves.

Equally important for your future is the increased self-esteem that you will have. Letting go of fear is an enormous challenge for everyone. Yet once you commit yourself to letting go of fear and take the first steps, each succeeding step becomes easier and before you know it, you feel lighter. Increased self-esteem gives you the physical and mental strength you need to take on other challenges associated with chronic illness.

The Nature of Fear

To let go of fear you first need to know what fear is. If you can recognize the different aspects of fears most commonly associated with chronic illness, you will better understand how your illness is affecting you. Fear is actually a complex emotional and physical phenomenon composed of different aspects, including *anxiety* and *phobias.*

Fear begins with a sense that something is threatening you. It might be a physical threat such as a nurse approaching you with a needle. It might be a psychological threat such as a phone call from the doctor saying that your recent colonoscopy showed an unusual growth. Or the threat can be both physical and psychological, such as an impending MRI that will involve spending up to an hour in a narrow, claustrophobia-inducing MRI tube while your ears are assaulted by loud clanging sounds.

Unfortunately, fear that comes from an actual experience like an MRI is self-reinforcing—the experience teaches you to fear other similar incidents or environments, like hospitals and doctors. But *anything that you learn can be unlearned.* Any fear can be modified or gotten rid of, if that is your desire. The effort required to let go of the fear associated with a threat will depend on how many times you have experienced the threat and the magnitude of the threat.

It is the nature of your mind that the strength of a threat experience will gradually diminish over time if you don't experience the same threat again. Repeated exposure to the same threat can embed the threat deeply in your memory so that the slightest appearance of the threat can bring about a very strong defensive response. Posttraumatic stress disorder (PTSD) is a fear response taken to its extreme. I once had an assistant who was a combat veteran. He experienced an artillery attack in which an incoming round exploded nearby and threw him across the bunker. Whenever he heard a loud noise at work, he would come into my office and sit nearby until his fear reaction subsided.

Fear is a basic survival tool that is deeply ingrained in human beings. Your mind and body have an automatic response of defending you against threats. You adjust the level of your defenses according to your estimate of the level of danger. Those defenses can work against you because they are unconscious and not necessarily in your best interests—your unconscious mind and your body are not really equipped to assess actual current situations and decide what to do about them. <u>The trick is to take conscious control of your fear response</u>.

A frequent companion of fear is **anxiety**. Perhaps you have experienced a fearful situation which caused you a great deal of anxiety. Your breathing quickened, your hands were soaked with sweat, and your heart pounded.

Your level of anxiety reflects your unconscious mind's assessment of your ability to cope with the threat. The greater your anxiety, the less confidence you have in your coping ability and the more likely you will flee instead of confronting the menace. On the other hand, if you are experiencing very little anxiety, you feel confident that you can successfully deal with the impending challenge.

It is very important for you to know that anxiety, like fear, is something that you can learn to control through knowledge and experience. Quite often, what seems to be an overwhelming situation that causes a great deal of anxiety is reduced to a manageable level once you understand the realities of the threat. The worksheet at the end of this chapter will show you how to do that. Shining the bright light of knowledge onto what is initially dark and menacing may reveal that it is really nothing to worry about. Your anxiety diminishes while your confidence increases.

For example, an invasive medical procedure that you've never experienced before may cause a great deal of anxiety. Because you have no prior experience with this procedure, your first goal is to learn as much as possible about it. This will allow you to put your arms around it and gain an understanding of the realities of the situation. Knowledge can help to reduce a threat to manageable dimensions. You can also benefit from the experience of others who have coped with your situation successfully. Medical and other support groups are invaluable and I urge you to join one.

Knowing what you are dealing with, combined with the experiences of others in the same situation, gives you tools for creating a plan for successfully coping with the anxiety-creating situation. Fear and anxiety move in tandem. As you gain control and reduce fear, your level of anxiety also decreases. Later in this chapter, I will show you how to manage and even conquer fear.

Phobias are another aspect of fear. A phobia is an irrational fear that goes way beyond the actual threat. A phobia may start out as a response to a potential threat, like germs or snakes, but the fear grows so large that the phobia — not germs or snakes — becomes disabling.

For example, it is quite reasonable and appropriate to protect yourself from an infectious disease. But a person who compulsively washes his hands after touching a doorknob has a germ phobia. He imagines that the germs on every doorknob are infectious and will make him very sick and maybe even kill him. A person with a phobia lives in a frightening and distorted world. The phobia becomes a prison that excludes many of the joys of life. <u>A phobia, like fear and anxiety, can be conquered</u>. If it is deeply rooted, the services of a therapist may be required.

Fears Related to Chronic Illness

There can be numerous fears associated with living just an ordinary and healthy (disease-free) life. Most people, most of the time, are able to keep their fears under control and carry on with their lives. When chronic illness strikes, old and new fears can overwhelm the mind. Here is a sample of the most common fears related to chronic illness:

- Making the wrong treatment decision
- Pain
- Death
- Invasive procedures (surgery, colonoscopy, CT scan, injection, biopsy, etc.)

- Financial ruin (impoverished by mounting medical bills)
- Being inferior to healthy people
- Loneliness or abandonment by family and friends
- Loss of control over body or mind (dementia, stroke)
- Being forced to adapt to a new and unwanted lifestyle (colostomy, checking blood sugar, insulin shots)
- Failure
- Criticism; ridicule
- Diminished physical capacity
- Loss of important lifelong leisure activities
- Never being able to fulfill your potential
- The unknown
- Loss of autonomy or freedom

Chronic illness can change your view of life and yourself. The onset and continued presence of chronic illness can make you pessimistic and fearful about your future. One specific fear may dominate your thoughts but others may also be present. Which fear concerns you most will depend on your life experiences and your fears before you became aware of your chronic illness. Also, different fears have greater impact at different stages of life.

Negative emotions, especially fear, can stop you in your tracks. Fear can freeze your mind and keep you from adapting to the physical and psychological changes brought about by your illness. At a time when you need to keep adapting to the endless stream of changes forced upon your body and mind, fear impairs your ability to adjust to those changes. Fear can envelop you like a thick fog, making it very hard to see where you are and where you need to go. The good news is that you can learn how to control your fears.

Good Fears and Bad Fears — Know the Difference

After hearing all the negative impacts that fear can have on you, it may be a surprise to learn that some types of fear are actually good for your health. Many people use the shock of their diagnosis and their fear of pain, disability, or death to make deep lifestyle changes to their diet, exercise, and stress levels. They get back on track and have a much better outcome than they would have had if fear had not jolted them out of their complacency. Notice that in this case these fears are realistic and should be heeded.

The fears that are not good for your health are those that involve psychological situations and conditions related to your chronic illness, especially fears that are greatly exaggerated. Unrealistic fears of dying, being abandoned, or disability — when they exceed the actual severity of your illness — are bad because they serve no positive protective purpose and they rob you of resources you need to take charge of your illness and your life.

The difference between a good fear and a bad fear is whether the fear can keep you out of harm's way (good fear) or endangers your well-being (bad fear). The former almost always refers to fears of physical suffering while the latter encompasses psychological fears.

Your Personal Fear Management Plan

Fear, anxiety, and phobias can be so strong that sometimes professional assistance is necessary to let go of them. If you feel you are in a fear crisis currently (for example, you are having severe anxiety attacks) or your fears are causing you significant depression, you should consider seeking out a therapist or other helping professional. Otherwise, I would like to encourage you to try to get your fears under control by thinking them through. Below is a worksheet that will guide you through each step of a process for understanding and eradicating your fears.

SELF-HELP FEAR-MANAGEMENT PLAN

For My Fears Related to _____

This worksheet will help you take a close look at your fears and work through them alone or with help. If you feel you need help, consider discussing your fear with a friend or family member, your doctor, a therapist, or a pastoral counselor. Often the presence of another person is enough to calm and clear your mind.

BEFORE YOU BEGIN

Before you begin working on this plan, make sure you are well rested and have eaten a healthy meal. Very often when you are tired, stressed, or hungry your anxiety rises, increasing your vulnerability to negative thoughts. Good physical care should precede any reflection you do about your chronic illness or your life situation.

STEP 1: GET CALM

Before you can think constructively about your fears, it's important to get calm. Choose one of these strategies, or find another one that will work for you:

- Slow breathing
- Meditation
- Listen to peaceful music
- Go for a walk in a calming environment
- Take a relaxing bath or shower
- Moderate exercise followed by a period of rest
- Go to your internal "sacred place" where you find peace and comfort

STEP 2: ACKNOWLEDGE YOUR FEARS & RATE THE INTENSITY OF EACH ONE ON A SCALE OF 1–10

1–2   Minimal
3–4   Moderately strong
5–6   Quite strong
7–8   Very strong
9–10   Extremely strong

FEAR   INTENSITY

1. _____

2. _____

3. _____

4. _____

STEP 3: UNDERSTAND YOUR FEARS

What is the current situation that is causing your fears?

How did these fears arise?

What is the reality of your situation, compared to your fears? Look at your situation calmly, as an external observer. What is the real level of threat to your well-being? Is the threat present right now?

What is the likelihood that your fears will come true if you take no action? When is that likely to happen?

If you were trying to help a friend who was in this situation, what would you say to help your friend understand the reality of the situation, as opposed to your friend's feelings of fear?

STEP 4: REFRAME YOUR THINKING IN A POSITIVE WAY

If your chronic illness is not curable, is it treatable? Would a successful treatment address some of your fears?

How much time do you have to find solutions?

What is good about your situation with respect to your illness and your life in general? For example, if one part of your body is not well, what parts or systems are functioning well? If you have lost some capacities, what things can you still do that are important to you?

Who is on your side now? Who cares about you? Who is working on your behalf? Who else can you contact for help?

What other resources do you have at this time? (Ways to get information, skills, financial resources, and so on)

Think about the insights and resources you have identified. How do those change your current situation and your future possibilities for the better?

STEP 5: STATE THE OUTCOMES YOU WANT FOR THE SITUATION THAT IS CAUSING YOUR FEARS

1.
2.
3.
4.
5.

STEP 6: MAKE AN ACTION PLAN

List the things you will do to get control of the situation that is causing your fears and achieve your desired outcome. Put them in order, starting with what you will do first. When you have finished this step, go back to Step 2 and check your level of anxiety again. Most likely you will note a significant drop in your anxiety by now.

1.

2.

3.

4.

5.

STEP 7: START WORKING ON YOUR PLAN

And KEEP working on it! You will find that each action you take will give you a greater sense of control over your situation, and your fears will subside as you work your way down your action list. All of those actions will accumulate and make a big dent in this thing that is causing your fear.

Despair

Despair is a state of deep hopelessness that happens when you feel overwhelmed by negative conditions and you see no solutions, no way out, no hope for the future. It can involve loss of your will and desire to live. When you sink that low, you stop caring about what happens. You may stop fighting your chronic illness and surrender to your darker thoughts, passivity, and self-pity. In that sense, despair can be lethal—more so than your chronic illness!

It is as if you're driving a car in the midst of rush-hour traffic and decide to take your hands off the steering wheel, close your eyes, and let the car go wherever the laws of physics take it. Eventually the car will crash into something or somebody. In like manner, a despairing person will ultimately crash physically and psychologically.

Many people with a chronic illness experience despair. Any serious illness potentially contains the seeds of despair in the very real conditions of the illness: fear of death; chronic pain from your illness or your treatment; feeling helpless and unable to cope; social isolation; and losses of all types, from your diminished physical capacities to your inability to work.

Learn to recognize these signs of despair that needs attention:

- Deep pessimism about everything, but especially your own life
- Passivity and malaise characterized by an attitude of "I don't care anymore"
- Being stubbornly committed to feeling hopeless; a rigid resistance to getting help or finding solutions
- Feeling sorry for yourself in a way that is debilitating
- Deliberate social isolation; keeping people at bay
- Seeking escape or relief through risky behaviors like alcohol abuse and unhealthy habits
- Loss of spiritual faith

Why Despair Is So Debilitating and Dangerous

You can understand despair by comparing it to its opposite: hope. Hope is an uplifting anticipation of good things to come in the future: the college acceptance letter, the long-awaited marriage proposal, the promotion at work. Hope brightens our view of the future. It buoys us up on the surface of life and keeps up optimistic no matter how many waves splash over us. It opens our mind to new opportunities and challenges. It puts us in a positive mood and receptiveness to others. *Hope is the basis of life!*

In the absence of hope, you can be alive but not have much life in you. Your heart beats; your lungs breathe; you walk, talk, eat, and so on. But without hope, you will lack the vitality of life. When you are in despair, you just go through the motions of living.

Despair is often associated with a real or perceived threat, like the fear of dying from a chronic illness. It's natural to want to flee from that threat. You are like an army that has lost its will to fight and is running away from the battlefield in a desperate scramble to get away at any cost. But the price you pay for not being able to face the enemy can be extreme physical and psychological stress. The threat doesn't go away just because you hide from it. It will always be in the back of your mind, adding fuel to your despair.

Despair is bad for your health in many ways. In order to fight your chronic illness, you need to be as healthy as possible both physically and psychologically. Continuous exposure to a high level of stress robs you of the resources and strength you need to direct against your illness. Despair not only weakens your defenses against your chronic illness, but also lowers your physical and mental resistance to other diseases.

Like many situations in life, it's hard to see a way out of despair when you're trapped in the middle of it. The way out is to shift your focus toward the things that can anchor and comfort you. That will get you to a place where you will be able to think about solutions to the problems that are causing your despair.

STEPS TO DEFEAT DESPAIR

STEP 1: GET HELP

Despair is a level of hopelessness that you might not be able to pull yourself out of without help. Talk with a family member, friend, therapist, or pastoral counselor. Choose a caring, accepting person who listens carefully to what you say and offers you comfort, insight, and helpful feedback. Seek professional help if talking to friends and family doesn't seem to be enough.

STEP 2: MAKE SURE YOU'RE BEING PROPERLY TREATED FOR PAIN

Pain can cloud your thinking and your judgment. There are remedies available for most types of pain. If your current remedy isn't working, talk to your doctor and make a workable pain-management plan.

STEP 3: TAKE CARE OF YOURSELF AND YOUR HOME ENVIRONMENT

Despair is reflected in the way you care for yourself and your home. Many people neglect their sleep, nutrition, personal hygiene, exercise, and their home when they're feeling despair. But being tired, hungry, and unshowered and in an untidy home reinforces the message that you're not in control of things. You can't clear your mind and solve problems in those conditions. They deenergize you and in fact increase your despair. Taking care of your basic physical needs and your home on a daily basis will give you a sense of control over your life. That will put you in a much better place mentally for thinking about the causes of your despair. Get help with any of these tasks that you can't do alone.

STEP 4: DEVELOP AN ACTION PLAN

Identify the causes of your despair and put them in order of priority. Make an action plan to address each problem. Begin working at the top of your list. You will be amazed at the power that taking action has to reverse despair and helplessness! *Action defeats despair.*

STEP 5: SEEK INSIGHT AND COMFORT IN YOUR FAITH

Your faith is there to comfort and serve you in your time of greatest need, which is now. Whatever your faith is, it connects you to greater forces beyond yourself and provides you with beliefs and insights that can sustain you now. Call on your faith now, and connect with fellow believers. Use your faith to understand the meaning of your present life situation. Ask for help. Shed your despair in prayer!

STEP 6: LIVE IN THE PRESENT MOMENT, ONE BREATH AT A TIME

Although your past and future may feel important to you, trying to live in the past, present, and future simultaneously is too much for anyone and will only increase your feelings of despair.

You may be especially worried about your future. It may feel like your illness has compromised your future. But there is a time for everything: a time for planning for the future; a time for taking action; a time for recovery. You're only one human being. You can really only be in one place at a time. You can only be taking action on one thing at a time. Once you've made a plan for solving a problem, ask yourself, "What is the ONE thing I can do about my situation at this present moment?" Then focus only on that ONE thing. Put your mind entirely into that one action. Don't allow your mind to drift into worries about the future or regrets about the past.

When you are stuck in worries about the future, you rob yourself of the potential peace and happiness of the present moment. Don't give away any hours or days of your life to the future or the past.

To test what I'm saying, close your eyes and try to empty your mind of all thoughts. Just let go of whatever thoughts, feelings, or images come into your mind. Notice that in this moment, absolutely nothing is being asked of you, except to just exist. Doesn't that feel wonderful? To only have to EXIST for a short time, in this present moment? Do this as often as you can throughout the day. You will notice a big shift in your despair. Your despair will move to the side as you come to cherish these simple moments of present existence.

Do each thing when it is time to do it. Go to the doctor when it is time. Be with your loved ones when it is time. Give your full attention to that one thing that you can do now, and let go of the dozens of things you can't do right now.

STEP 7: MAKE TIME FOR HAPPINESS EACH AND EVERY DAY

Your daily schedule probably includes tasks like appointments, errands, and many other things you must do. I would like you to add a box to your schedule for pleasurable activities. Draw up a list of all the things you find pleasurable, things that make you smile and laugh and bring you serenity: being with friends and family, music, reading, watching a movie, day trips, and so on. Choose at least one thing from this list each day and write it on your schedule. <u>Treat this activity as just as important as everything else on your schedule</u>, not as something optional or unnecessary. Your pleasure activities will renew your emotional, spiritual, physical, and mental energy, making you stronger for the next actions you need to take to address your illness.

What if you just don't feel like doing anything pleasurable? <u>Do it anyway</u>. Act as if you were happy. Ask yourself, "If I were happy, how would I spend this day?" Then do that. If you incorporate pleasure into your daily routine, it will soon become a habit and you will experience real improvement in your mood and feelings of hope.

Anger

Does your chronic illness sometimes make you angry? Many people come to deeply resent the limitations imposed by their illness — you can no longer do all that you used to do. Moments of annoyance, irritation, and even anger can accompany the many issues that arise with chronic illness. Perhaps it's trying to keep track of the endless number of appointments with different doctors and therapists. Or it might be your frustration with arriving on time for an appointment and then having to wait half an hour without any explanation for the delay. Chronic pain can turn a previously easygoing personality into an irritated and constantly complaining grouch.

Anger is a natural defense mechanism that is a part of the fight-or-flight response. Eons ago, the purpose of this response was to protect us against attacks from predators or other sources of physical harm. In modern life, however, humans have adapted the fight-or-flight response to include perceived or actual psychological and physical threats.

The Dimensions of Anger

Anger has three basic dimensions: frequency, intensity, and memories of past events. When the nurse or doctor wants to know how much pain you're experiencing, you will be asked, "On a scale of 1 to 10, where 10 is the worst pain you've ever experienced, how much pain are you feeling now?" You can rate the intensity of your anger in the same way. You can be slightly angry (annoyed), somewhat angry (irritated), seething mad (really angry), or somewhere in between any of these points. Anger is like the temperature of running water: cool, tepid, warm, hot, or boiling.

Answering the following questions will help you understand your anger temperament and whether or not you need to adjust how you react to events and people.

- How often do you get angry? *Infrequently, occasionally, frequently,* or *daily*?
- When you get angry, are you usually *annoyed, irritated,* or *really mad*?
- Is there *some specific situation or person* that makes you intensely angry?

How big is the box of anger that you carry around with you, ready to respond to situations that irritate you? If it is out of proportion to events or is causing you problems, you need to make it smaller. It may be helpful for you to know that it is possible to change your response to the things that aggravate and frustrate you, to reduce the frequency and intensity of your anger episodes.

Controlling Anger Is Essential for Your Health

Chronic, intense anger is a very toxic emotion that can directly cause illnesses like heart disease and possibly even cancer. It is believed to impact the body right down to the cellular level. Anger poisons the mind and body. It sets up an overall negative physical and mental disposition that is not conducive to health or happiness.

Here are some of the negative aspects of anger that are harmful to your health:

- Anger can rob you of valuable energy your body and mind need for fighting your chronic illness.
- Anger increases your stress level, which can damage your immune system—your vital defense against disease. You already have a chronic illness—why would you knowingly encourage other diseases to invade your body?
- Anger is toxic to relationships. It makes you find fault with people and hold grudges. It can create a desire for revenge, which only leads to more anger.
- Anger can isolate you from people who could be important members of your chronic illness support team. Strong, long-held grudges create barriers over time that become very difficult to overcome ("I haven't spoken to my father or mother in years").
- Happy, pleasant people do not want to be around an angry person, so angry people tend to associate with other angry people.
- Anger can be addictive. There are some people who seek the thrill of danger and the stimulation created by turning on the fight-or-flight response. Strong anger responses can bring forth an adrenaline high.
- Anger can create a false sense of self-righteousness and esteem. Angry people do not like to hear contrary opinions or facts. They prefer to surround themselves with a self-created atmosphere that supports their anger. That closes them off to the information they need for well-being.

Strategies for Dealing with Short-Term Anger

Short-term anger is like a food or wine stain on your clothing: the sooner you act to remove it from the fabric of your life, the easier it is to get rid of it. The longer you allow it to remain, the more stubborn and resistant it becomes to removal. Listed below are several "stain removers" that can be quite successful in helping you get rid of short-term anger. Which one is best for you will depend on the situation, your personality, and — most important of all — your desire to rid yourself of anger.

Live in the present. This is a very effective method for overcoming short-term anger because all your energies, thoughts, and actions are focused on Now. You don't allow your mind to consider anything negative from the past: events, people, or emotions. Living in the present means that your mind and body are concentrating on what you need and should be doing at this very moment.

Listen and learn from the experiences of others. There are many frustrating experiences that are common among people with a chronic illness. It can be very helpful to learn how others have coped successfully with their own frustrations and anger through a support group, reading and research, and Internet forums. Tapping into the experiences and reactions of others can open your eyes and mind to your options for ridding yourself of burdensome anger.

Change the situation. It may be that a specific and recurring situation is causing your anger. Perhaps you feel that the receptionist at your doctor's office is rude to you whenever you arrive for an appointment. You can change the situation by talking to the receptionist, the office manager (if there is one), or your doctor about how you are being treated by the receptionist. Discussing the situation can resolve the problem and allow you to shed your anger.

Learn to forgive. To forgive someone for their actions is your choice and not theirs. It is easy to say, "I forgive someone for what has been done to me." However, true forgiveness is a challenging process that can only be achieved over time. Every major religion addresses the issue of forgiveness, because true forgiveness is truly healing. Forgiveness is best used for resolving major causes of anger and not minor incidents of irritation.

Laughter. Humor is like a laundry detergent. It can remove the stains of anger and brighten your life. Be sure to follow the directions on the package. As a patient once said, "After twenty years of therapy my psychiatrist said something that brought tears to my eyes. He said, 'No hablo ingles.'"[2]

Change your view of life. For most people, changing their view of life is quite a challenge. We like familiar surroundings, including the way we see ourselves, our friends and family, and everything else in the world. Once you have created an image of someone, you find it very annoying to be told that your image is out of date, that it doesn't match reality. It is common to hear senior citizens complain, "Things were much better when I was young" or "The older days were better." That only means that they prefer the familiar and have difficulty adjusting to an unfamiliar world.

A chronic illness has all the ingredients to set you up with a long-term negative view of things: pain, diminishing capacities, invasive medical procedures, and so on. If you allow your attention and your energy to be absorbed by those, your anger will only increase. Choose instead to shift your attention to all the things that are going <u>right</u> in your life and all that you have. Adopt an automatic attitude of gratitude. If you hear a voice in the back of your mind saying, "I HATE going to these appointments!" speak back to it firmly and say, "I'm so grateful that I have access to medical care that can ease my pain."

This metaphor, told to me by Reverend Frederick Nyanguf, may help you let go of short-term anger: "Anger is like holding a butterfly in your hand. You can vent your anger on the butterfly by crushing it in your hand. The result will be a mess that you will have to clean up. Or you can open your hand and free the butterfly. As it flies away, your eyes will follow as it leads you to see the beauty of the world around you."

Dealing with Long-Term Anger and Grudges

Long-term anger is toxic to your mind and body. It is particularly harmful to anyone with a chronic illness — someone who needs to be as healthy as possible. The average patient understands the importance of avoiding anything that is harmful to health, especially something toxic. Yet otherwise reasonable people deliberately expend valuable strength, energy, and time maintaining long-held memories of experiences and people that have aroused strong feelings of anger in the past. Why do they do that?

Those feelings are addictive. They initiate a strong fight reaction with no thought of flight. Anger gives vent to desires and fantasies of revenge. Strong, long-held anger can feed on itself to create even greater anger until it becomes rage. Rage creates a sense of power directed at gaining vengeance against the source of the anger, whoever or whatever it may be.

Do you have a long-held anger that, once aroused, is hard to contain and control? Is there someone toward whom you hold a grudge? Is there someone that you won't speak to because of your anger? If any of these conditions apply to you, you should seek professional counseling to rid yourself of long- and strongly held feelings of anger, because they may be causing great harm to your health.

Shame and Guilt

Shame and guilt can come from events in your past or stem directly from your chronic illness. In either case, they are strong negative emotions that you should remove from your baggage in order to have greater emotional freedom and health.

People commonly think of shame and guilt as variations of the same negative emotion, differing only in intensity. They do share some common features. For example, shame and guilt are both responses to specific events, often involving other people. The result of these events can cause you to have a negative self-image.

However, extensive psychological research has shown that shame and guilt are entirely different emotions. They have different origins, which bring about very different personal behaviors.

Shame

Shame causes a person to feel inadequate, incapable, or inferior compared to other people. Shame is about how you feel about *yourself*. It can be either externally imposed or self-created. In the first instance, it can be the result of efforts of parents, teachers, employers, and other authority figures to discipline or control someone by making unfavorable comparisons to others.

"You're being very bad. Good children don't wet their bed."

"The coach makes me sit on the bench and won't let me play at any of the games. He says I'm the worst member on the team and he just keeps me around to motivate the other players."

"Everyone in the office got a raise this year except me. My boss said my sales were the lowest he's ever seen."

Often some form of punishment follows the effort to cause shame.

Shame can be self-created when you compare yourself to someone else and conclude that you are inferior in some way: "I'm the only person in my family who didn't go to college." "My brothers and sisters all earn much more than I do."

Shame, regardless of how it was created, can adversely affect your health in several ways. First, it darkens your self-image. You may come to see yourself as inferior, incomplete, or incompetent. You feel that you are just not as good as others. Shame can cause you to focus only on your shortcomings—which may or may not be as bad as you think, or even real. However, what you perceive about yourself determines how you behave, because perception is reality.

Shame creates a sense of permanent inferiority and erodes your self-confidence. "I've failed at most things in life. I just don't have what it takes to succeed." Shame wounds the mind and causes a great deal of emotional pain.

No one wants to be shamed. You might think that it feels better to stand in the shadows of society, where you're not seen, rather than in the light, where a shortcoming might be revealed. Sometimes shame is so powerful that it causes you to react aggressively or deny your personal responsibility for your actions.

If the origin of your shame is a sense of personal unworthiness, it is possible to overcome that negative emotion by turning your attention to your positive qualities: things that you do well, positive personality traits. Everyone can do something well. Everyone has positive personal traits. If you focus all your energies on using your skills and presenting your positive qualities, you won't have any energy left for dwelling on your shame and it will eventually fade.

With respect to chronic illness, the most common and greatest source of shame is the sense of being less capable than before. You want to do the things you used to do so easily, but now find them difficult or impossible. You may feel that it's your fault that you have lost certain capacities.

"I use to be a walking encyclopedia. Now I have such a hard time remembering things."

"Before my illness, using the computer was effortless. Now, it takes forever just to answer one e-mail because my hands shake so much. I feel so incompetent."

"I feel like such a burden on my friends and family. I can no longer take care of myself. They have to do so much for me."

"It's getting harder and harder to speak clearly. People have a hard time understanding what I'm saying. It's so embarrassing."

I recommend that you offer yourself the acceptance and compassion that you hope to receive from others relative to your illness. Instead of feeling ashamed of what you have lost or can no longer do, be who you are with pride, and do what you can do with pride.

It is possible to overcome shame and transform yourself. However, it is hard work and takes time and motivation. If a sense of shame is deeply embedded in your personality, professional counseling may help you.

Guilt

Guilt is very different from shame. Shame creates a negative attitude toward yourself. Shame is like a shroud that covers all of you and causes you to feel unworthy.

Guilt, on the other hand, is focused on a specific behavior, on something you did that you believe was wrong. Guilt leads you to say, "That was not a good thing I did." Guilt is often the result of violating some rule of society, or your own personal values and standards.

A chronic illness demands so much of you. That can come to feel like a burden. Not only are you having difficulty doing the things you used to do, but now you have a new set of doctor's orders to follow. Many people feel guilty when they are unable to do all of those tasks to perfection — doing all the physical therapy exercises every day; taking all the right pills at the right time; following a new diet; monitoring your blood sugar regularly.

And of course, you may also feel guilty about your past behaviors that contributed to your chronic illness. Did you ignore the warning signs of your illness? Not listen when your doctor told you to change your diet, exercise more, and stop smoking or suffer the consequences? Now your illness has affected not only your life, but also the lives of your family and friends.

When guilt is out of proportion to its cause, lasts for months or years, or causes you suffering, it is unhealthy and needs to be resolved. Resolving guilt is not easy when you have actually done something that you know was wrong. To acknowledge your personal failure can feel like a hurdle that is too high to overcome. But if you are willing to rid yourself of guilt, you will find that the emotional effort of admitting guilt is easier than the effort of concealing and denying it.

Often people feel guilty about things they actually weren't responsible for. Perhaps you did your best as a parent, with the resources you had at the time, and yet your adult child faults you. Own up to your past shortcomings and whatever harm you actually caused, but don't allow other people to magnify your responsibility beyond what actually occurred. Dialog with the people involved will help you make amends and find closure.

We usually think of guilt as a negative emotion. But it is an amazing fact that guilt can help you become healthier! Guilt focuses your attention on a specific action that you did. In your guilt, you acknowledge that this was something you should not have done. Guilt is a positive force if it makes you want to make amends for that inappropriate behavior and not do it again.

Guilt involving other people can be a positive factor in your life when three conditions are met:

1. You acknowledge and take personal responsibility for your actions.
2. You make a commitment (a promise, a vow) to not repeat the offending action.
3. You make amends for what you did. This could be in the form of an apology or some kind of compensation to people you have harmed.

In some religions, such as Judaism, Christianity, and Islam, inappropriate behavior is called "sin." In other religions, such as Buddhism and Shinto, and the secular world, behavior that causes guilt is considered a violation of a code of ethics.

Whether you call inappropriate actions sin or unethical acts, it is a good outcome when guilt causes you to improve your behavior. If you act on your guilt and change your behavior, significant changes will occur. Your self-image and self-respect will improve, your stress level will decrease, and even your physical appearance will improve. All these changes are beneficial to your health.

Resolution of shame and guilt can lead you to act in a more caring, responsible, and positive manner toward others, and especially toward yourself. Ridding yourself of the heavy emotional baggage of shame and guilt will bring you strength and courage to fight your chronic illness.

Emotional Baggage and Faith

What Is Faith?

Does the word "faith" raise your hackles, increase your stress level, or make you angry? Some people bristle at the mention of faith. To them, faith is the same as religion. Just mention faith and they are reminded of distasteful and unhappy religious experiences that occurred at some time in their past or are occurring even now. Let me assure you that the brief discussion of faith here and the in-depth discussion in part 4 are focused on helping you to achieve peace and meaning in your life. You will bring to our discussion a personal definition of faith that is based on your view of life.

Faith, as defined and used in this book, includes two things:

1. A belief that gives meaning to your life
2. Incorporating your belief in everything you do

This is a faith that you have created for yourself and it has the power to sustain you in times of despair and suffering.

Faith Is Important to Your Well-Being

Living with a chronic illness has its good and bad moments. The longer you live with a chronic illness, the more the bad moments can begin to weigh you down. As time passes, it can get harder to bounce back from the difficult moments. It is exactly at these times that faith can help you. A strong faith has many benefits:

- Faith gives you physical and mental strength.
- Faith gives direction to your life.
- Faith gives you resolve.
- Faith gives you hope.
- Faith connects you to a greater presence beyond yourself.

Chronic illness can damage or even destroy your faith. By its very nature and definition, chronic illness has become a permanent part of your life. It is not going away, and it keeps changing. Physical and mental suffering have become your constant companions. The need to continually adjust your life to the demands of your illness can wear you down and erode your faith. As your faith diminishes, so does hope. The loss of faith can be particularly troubling if your faith is founded on a belief in a benevolent and personal God. You may feel that God has abandoned you in your greatest time of need.

The focus of this chapter is on helping you to let go of your negative emotional baggage. Removing those emotions makes room for a positive faith. In part 4, we will discuss in depth how to develop your own personal faith that is uplifting and will sustain you at all times, good and bad.

CHAPTER 5

Overcoming Loneliness

BEING ALONE OR FEELING ALONE is one of the most painful conditions that a human being can experience. It can have profound consequences for your mental and physical health. Many people feel trapped in loneliness and don't know how to make the connections they need with other people. It can be especially difficult to maintain old connections and make new ones when you're dealing with a chronic illness. In this chapter we will explore why those connections are especially important for you during your chronic illness and what you can do to strengthen them.

We All Need People

Instinctively, people seek to live together in groups, which may have as few as two people or may number in the thousands and millions. Biologically speaking, the purpose of forming close bonds with others is to increase our chances of obtaining the basic needs of life: food, water, shelter from the elements, clothing, and personal safety. But our need for people goes much deeper than that. It is at the root of every aspect of our well-being: our happiness, our optimism about the future, our feeling that we have control over our fate and that we have allies as we face life's biggest challenges. Relationships are not only about the support we receive from others — they also allow us to have a sense of purpose through what we give to others. A person who feels alone or who is truly alone loses the spark of life that is needed to keep moving forward in good times and in bad.

Dr. Martin Seligman, a leading authority on the new science called Positive Psychology, has developed an understanding of how people stay mentally healthy that he calls the Well-Being Theory.[3] His research has found that five factors are important for good mental health:

1. Positive emotion
2. Engagement
3. Meaning
4. Achievement
5. Relationships

In my experience providing pastoral counseling to patients, I find that establishing and maintaining meaningful relationships with other people is the most critical of these components.

Meaningful relationships can take many forms: friendship, marriage, family, coworkers, activity groups, volunteer work, and so on. Friends are particularly important throughout the lifespan. People become friends because each one benefits psychologically from knowing the other and sharing common experiences. Over time, friends develop together a "language of experiences" that is unique to their friendship and requires very little use of spoken words. Everyone needs to have at least one friend like this.

Loneliness is an unfulfilled desire for the presence and company of other people. This yearning can be for someone specific such as a good friend or a loved one who has died. Or it can be for a group of friends who have shared important experiences with you and used to meet regularly but no longer do so because of finances, distance, or age. Or it can be a longing for family.

The absence of at least one meaningful relationship, or the loss of a loved one or a very special friendship which may have lasted for years or decades, can bring about a deep sense of isolation from society, grief, and a yearning for connections with others. If you remain alone or lonely for too long, it can severely impact your health and result in depression. However, *loneliness is reversible*. In this chapter, I will show you how to combat loneliness and develop new friendships which can, over time, become very meaningful.

It's Good to Be Alone at Times — But Not All the Time

Sometimes you need peace and quiet away from others and from the stresses of your illness, time when you can focus only on your own needs or interests, gather your thoughts, or heal emotionally, physically, or spiritually. These precious moments of chosen solitude can be very beneficial, and I encourage you to create quality time alone.

On the other hand, solitude that you don't choose for yourself can be quite detrimental. Many people slide into loneliness without realizing it, and for the wrong reasons, including the negative emotions associated with a chronic illness, such as anger, fear, shame, embarrassment, or depression. In these instances, solitude is not beneficial for you.

Loneliness Is Bad for Your Health

As Mother Theresa said, "The most terrible poverty is loneliness, and the feeling of being unloved." Don't underestimate the importance of having good connections with people. You need people as much as you need the other basics of life. Loneliness can cause great mental anguish that darkens your view of yourself and the future. You see yourself in terms of your limitations and begin to believe that other people see you the same way.

Loneliness can bring about great sadness, depression, and loss of hope. Your vitality diminishes. Many people who are alone feel such a loss of energy and hope that they begin to neglect themselves with respect to nutrition, hygiene and appearance, healthcare, their home, and their responsibilities. Self-neglect only drives you deeper into isolation.

Last but certainly not least, being alone can impair the immune system, which chronically ill people cannot afford.

Research has shown that positive relationships boost the immune system.

Why Chronically Ill People Are Often Lonely

We have seen in previous chapters that a chronic illness can bring major changes to your life and even who you are as a person. Other people perceive those changes, and they may have difficulty adjusting to them. Perhaps they feel that you are no longer the person they used to know.

A common cause of loneliness for someone with a chronic illness is that family and friends may turn away from you, perhaps unintentionally. They no longer communicate with you by telephone, e-mail, or letters. They don't visit you as they did in the past. They don't include you in their social activities. It may feel to you that people are acting as if you no longer exist!

Your illness may have reduced your capabilities so that you cannot participate fully in activities as you once did. For example, if you have difficulty walking, your hiking friends no longer include you in their hikes. Perhaps some of your friends feel you've changed so much that you no longer fit into their social network.

Some people feel very awkward in the presence of a person with an illness. They focus on your illness and not on the relationship that existed before you became ill. You remind them of their own vulnerability and mortality, which makes them uncomfortable. They don't know what to say to you or what to talk about. They are concerned that they will offend you by focusing on your illness. Initially, they may try to pretend that you are not chronically ill. Eventually, the effort becomes tiring and they just turn away from you.

Your illness is ever present to you and unconsciously, it may come up frequently in conversation. This is particularly true among senior citizens. It's likely that continually hearing about the details of a person's ailments, doctors, and medications will alienate others.

The above explanations for loneliness are about other people's behaviors toward a chronically ill person. But loneliness is a two-sided coin, and there are things that make chronically ill people turn away from their family, friends, and acquaintances. Distancing yourself from others can be a deliberate action, or sometimes you just slip away from those who once were an important part of your life. It's important to become aware of how you are maintaining your relationships. Perhaps you can relate to some of these situations that limit relationships for people with a chronic illness:

- You are ashamed or embarrassed that you are chronically ill. You think that people see you as something less than what you were before, regardless of whether this is true or not. *Antidote*: Don't overidentify with your illness. You are more than your illness. Present yourself as a whole person.
- You tire more easily. You have less energy for social activities with friends and family. *Antidote*: Learn to manage your energy by alternating periods of activity and rest, and with good physical care.

- Your circle of acquaintances is getting smaller every year. As you age, inevitably friends die and sometimes they aren't replaced. *Antidote*: Form new friendships.
- Your interests have changed or diminished. Things that interested you before don't have much appeal anymore. *Antidote*: Pursue the activities that still interest you and develop new ones.
- You're less interested in what is going on in your community, the nation, or the world. You have withdrawn from the world. You have become more focused on just yourself. *Antidote*: Get outside yourself. Turn your focus outward. Take steps to become more involved with the world.
- You haven't been able to come to terms with your illness emotionally and are experiencing feelings of depression, grief, and loss. *Antidote*: Isolation will only increase those feelings. Restore balance to your life by cultivating positive relationships and being as active as you can. Work through your feelings about your illness with a counselor if necessary.

Ways to Overcome Loneliness

Making new friends can be difficult even for healthy people, especially as they age and lose old friends. Regardless of the cause of your loneliness, you may find that you have fewer and fewer contacts with people who share your interests. It is as if you had a fruit tree in your front yard that provided you with an abundance of very fine fruit for many years but is no longer productive. The time has come for you to plant a new tree and nurture it until it begins to bear fruit for you.

The more people you meet, the better your chances of making one or more new friends. Below are some ideas for things you can do to increase your possibilities of making new friends and building quality relationships.

1. Create Peaceful and Meaningful Solitude

I place this first because happiness starts within, and the best relationships happen when you are at peace with yourself regardless of your present condition or circumstances. Above I mentioned the positive benefits of time spent alone, when you are quietly recharging your batteries after taking care of your responsibilities.

What will you do during your self-chosen solitude? Think about what is uplifting and restorative for you. Some possibilities:

- Meditation, prayer, or quiet contemplation
- Time spent in nature
- Soothing outdoor activities like walking, biking, or kayaking done at a leisurely pace
- Any other activity that you enjoy: reading, writing, listening to or playing music, artwork, hobbies, watching old movies

Use this time to learn to be content with yourself and to create positive thoughts and feelings to counterbalance any negative emotions associated with your chronic illness. Practice being in the present moment, focusing only on your chosen activity and letting go of all worries about your illness and concerns about the future.

When you have learned to be alone peacefully you may be surprised to find that people will be drawn to your positive mental state.

2. Get a Pet

A pet offers several benefits to everyone, not just the lonely. A pet can be a loving and devoted companion to a person who lives alone. Taking care of a pet can make you feel that you have a purpose in life as the animal depends on you for its well-being.

Walking a dog every day is great for your health, and it can offer the additional benefit of interaction with the people you meet on your walk, especially if your dog is well-behaved, well-groomed, and friendly.

If you're thinking of getting a pet please carefully consider what that will entail. Your pet will need your daily presence and attention, which can limit your freedom. If you want to go away for a few days you will need to find someone to care for your pet while you are away. Also think about the cost of a pet's food, medical care, and other needs. Walking and grooming a dog can be physically demanding.

If you feel you can handle the responsibilities of taking care of an animal, having a pet might bring needed companionship and love into your life.

The 2008 movie *Gran Torino*, featuring Clint Eastwood, dramatically portrays the relation between solitude based on negative emotions and loneliness, the role of pet companion-ship, and how friendship brings meaning to life. If you are lonely, you might gain some insights by watching this film.

3. Choose Face-to-Face Contact with People

If your loneliness is the result of inadequate interaction with others, the antidote is to increase your contact with peo-ple. The greater the number of new people you come in con-tact with, the greater the chances that you'll find someone who becomes a friend. Usually it takes more than one conversation with someone to establish the beginnings of mutual interests and understanding.

Face-to-face communication is the best way to establish a relationship. When you are speaking with someone directly, much of the information communicated between you and the other person is nonverbal, transmitted by body language — the facial and other body gestures that provide the emotional framework for what is said. For example, folded arms are a strong signal that the other person is rejecting what you are saying or what you stand for. Arms spread apart are a sign of welcome and receptiveness. Have you ever been hugged by someone with folded arms?

Interaction that is not face-to-face can be misleading because you are deprived of critical nonverbal information that you need in order to accurately understand the other per-son's message and to judge the truth of what is being said to you. If you are speaking to someone on the telephone who says, "That's a really good idea," you don't have the benefit of nonverbal information to decide whether the other person really likes your idea or is privately grimacing at the thought of your suggestion. E-mail and text messages are even less reliable vehicles of personal and meaningful communication even if you know the other person relatively well. Face-to-face contact with people is simply more satisfying and "real."

4. Use Modern Social Technology

Having said that face-to-face relationships are best, I recognize that many people live in rural areas where their opportunities for direct contact with others may be limited, and at times a chronic illness can make it difficult to get out and see people. If that's your case, use the telephone, e-mail, Facebook, a web camera on your computer, or whatever other means work for you to be in touch with people. In this day and age you can live in a small town in Alaska and be in contact literally with people around the globe.

5. Volunteer

One of the best ways to meet new people is to become a volunteer for an organization that matches your interests and skills. Volunteerism is the backbone of American culture. From the earliest days of the first British settlements in North America, neighbors pitched in to help each other with tasks too large for one person to accomplish, like building homes, clearing fields, and harvesting crops. George Washington, Benjamin Franklin, and most other leaders of the young United States were members of a volunteer fire company. Today, nearly every nonprofit organization throughout the United States—hospitals, libraries, schools, parks, municipal recreational facilities, and museums—depends upon the work of volunteers to carry out its service mission.

If you want to have a successful volunteer experience that results in enjoyable and pleasant interactions with other members of the staff, you need to do some homework and planning before you contact organizations. There are two important questions to consider:

First, *what kind of volunteer experience are you looking for?* You may have a special interest, a hobby, or a particular skill that you can share with others through volunteer work. You can also develop your knowledge in a particular area as a volunteer. If you enjoy history, there is undoubtedly a local historical society or museum near you. If you enjoy reading, every community has a public library that uses volunteers in many different roles. A support group for your chronic illness may have an office near you that needs your organizational help. Volunteer opportunities are limited only by your imagination.

Second, *what kind of volunteers is the organization looking for?* The size and specialty of an organization are important factors in determining which volunteer roles are available. Volunteer opportunities start with entry-level responsibilities that require little or no experience or training. Often you will receive training on the job for relatively simple work like sorting canned goods in a food pantry or answering questions at a hospital information desk.

At the next level are volunteer positions that require some prior training or related experience that is beneficial to the organization's mission and activities.

At the highest level of volunteering are professional opportunities that require a relatively high level of training, experience, and expertise. For example, a volunteer museum docent who gives talks to groups of visitors about an exhibit will be expected to be a good public speaker and have knowledge of the museum's areas of interest.

The organization you volunteer for will invest its resources in you with additional training to make you a valued member of the staff. Most often, the organization will require a minimum commitment of time and effort from you in exchange for the training or other benefits you receive.

Don't forget that the objective of being a volunteer in an organization is to increase your contact with people. So make a point of seeking volunteer work that will allow you to spend time with people rather than solitary work. The worksheet at the end of this chapter will help you figure out what volunteer opportunity would be a good fit for you.

6. Connect with People Who Share Your Interests

One of the best ways to do this is to join an activity group. These days there are groups and clubs for virtually every interest and hobby imaginable. Use the Internet and your local newspaper to find a group to join.

7. Be Brave: Practice Your Conversation Skills

Watch for opportunities to reach out in conversation to people wherever you go. This involves some personal emotional risk so you will need to move beyond your present comfort zone, but you may be rewarded with a new friendship.

8. Extend Invitations to People

To learn more about your new acquaintances and for them to become acquainted with you, create small social occasions such as having a cup of coffee or lunch together or attending a cultural event or other activity that you're both interested in.

9. Stay in Touch

Make an effort to regularly stay in contact with people whose company you enjoy. Make a point of spending time with at least one friend every week.

10. Join a Support Group

If you feel that your friendships have dwindled as a direct result of your chronic illness, it may help you to share those feelings with others who have a similar illness and learn from them how they manage to stay connected in spite of their illness. You may find new friendships in a support group.

11. Join a Faith Community

A faith organization brings together people with common beliefs and values. Many religious organizations offer activities and volunteer opportunities that go well beyond the weekly service.

12. Look Up Old Friends

These days finding old friends is quite easy using the Internet. You may be surprised to find that friends from long ago are glad to hear from you.

Developing and maintaining relationships is an on-going endeavor. It requires your continuing attention to be successful but is well worth the effort to overcome loneliness. Be inspired by this quote from Albert Schweitzer that reminds us of the importance of being connected:

> In everyone's life, at some time, our inner fire goes out. It is then burst into flame by an encounter with another human being. We should all be thankful for those people who rekindle the inner spirit.

WORKSHEET #1

MY PLAN TO INCREASE MY CONNECTIONS

STEP 1: WHAT IS THE CURRENT STATE OF YOUR RELATIONSHIPS?

1   I have no close relationships and I feel deeply lonely. I feel withdrawn from the world.

2   I have a couple of acquaintances or family members I see occasionally, but no real close friend I can confide in.

3   I have one close friend and/or am close to one or more family members.

4   I have a few or several close friends, associates, and/or family members who I spend time with fairly often.

5   My relationships bring me the love, support, and stimulation I need, and I have opportunities to offer love and support to others, including in my paid work or volunteer work. I am actively involved in the world.

STEP 2: CREATE MEANINGFUL TIME ALONE.

How I will spend my time alone:

1. _____
2. _____
3. _____
4. _____

STEP 3: WHAT TYPES OF RELATIONSHIPS DO YOU WANT TO INCREASE OR ENHANCE?

___ Contact with family members

___ Maintain current friendships

___ Make new friends

___ Volunteer work

___ Activity partners

___ People who share my interest in _____

___ People who have my chronic illness

___ People who share my religious or spiritual beliefs

___ Involvement in social and political causes: _____

___ Animals

___ Other:_____

STEP 4: CREATE A PLAN FOR EACH TYPE OF RELATIONSHIP YOU WANT TO INCREASE OR ENHANCE

List all the ideas you can think of to increase each type of relationship you identified above.

TYPE OF RELATIONSHIP, HOW I CAN INCREASE OR ENHANCE IT

1. _____

2. _____

3. _____

4. _____

5. _____

6. _____

STEP 5: BEGIN IMPLEMENTING YOUR PLAN

WORKSHEET #2

BECOMING A VOLUNTEER

STEP 1: INVENTORY WHAT YOU CAN BRING TO AN ORGANIZATION

MY INTERESTS AND HOBBIES

1. _____
2. _____
3. _____
4. _____
5. _____

MY SKILLS, TALENTS, AND PERSONAL QUALITIES

1. _____
2. _____
3. _____
4. _____
5. _____

MY TRAINING

1. _____
2. _____
3. _____
4. _____
5. _____

MY EXPERIENCE

1. _____

2. _____

3. _____

4. _____

5. _____

STEP 2: IDENTIFY THE QUALITIES OF A SUCCESSFUL VOLUNTEER EXPERIENCE FOR YOU

1. What specific interests, skills, and experience do you want to apply in a volunteer capacity?

   1. _____

   2. _____

   3. _____

   4. _____

   5. _____

2. What level of work do you want to perform?

   ___ Entry level

   ___ Semi-skilled

   ___ Professional

3. Do you want to learn new skills?   YES   NO

4. How much time do you want to give to volunteer work each week or each month?

   _____

5. Are you willing to make a long-term commitment to an organization, such as two hours a week for one

year? What time commitment would you be comfortable making?

_____

6. Would you like to work for a small or a large organization, or doesn't it matter?

    In a small nonprofit organization, you will get to know everyone, from the president to the maintenance person. In a very large organization with more than one hundred volunteers, like a large urban hospital, you may become acquainted with only a few staff members and some volunteers.

    _____

7. Does your chronic illness limit the kind of volunteer work you can participate in? How?

    _____

8. Considering your answers to the above questions, describe your ideal volunteer experience.

    Type of organization:_____

    Size: _____

    My duties: _____

    My schedule: _____

    My working conditions: _____

STEP 3: CONTACT ORGANIZATIONS THAT MIGHT MATCH YOUR IDEAL VOLUNTEER EXPERIENCE

ORGANIZATION   CONTACT PERSON, PHONE #

1. _____

2. _____

3. _____

4. _____

5. _____

QUESTIONS I WANT TO ASK EACH ORGANIZATION:

1. _____

2. _____

3. _____

4. _____

5. _____

STEP 4: MEET WITH EACH ORGANIZATION, AND CHOOSE THE ONE THAT BEST FITS YOUR IDEAL VOLUNTEER EXPERIENCE

Clarify what your duties, schedule, and other working conditions would be. Ask to tour the facility and meet with some of the staff and volunteers.

STEP 5: EVALUATE YOUR EXPERIENCE AFTER 3 TO 4 MONTHS OF VOLUNTEERING

Do you enjoy being a volunteer at this organization? If not, talk with the volunteer manager about your experience to date and how it might be improved.

Give the experience a chance to succeed. It takes time and patience for a volunteer to fit into the culture of any organization. Think about ways you can adapt to the organization to make your time there easier and more productive.

Which of these strategies would improve your volunteer experience?

___ Greet people with a smile

___ Take time to socialize with people, even for just a minute

___ Show interest in learning about each person you meet. Try to remember the person's name and one fact about the person. Keep a list of people you have frequent interaction with.

___ Minimize talking about yourself but be open to sharing information about yourself if it will enrich a conversation.

___ Avoid talking about your illness.

___ Be open to learning new skills and ways of doing things.

___ Remember to enjoy yourself.

___ Other strategies: _____

Part 3

FIND NEW MEANING IN LIFE

CHAPTER 6

Change Your Perspective
to Live a Larger Life

Unmet Expectations

I USED TO WORK AS an EMT. One afternoon I was finishing the paperwork on a patient we had just brought into the emergency department when I was startled by a medical team rushing past me toward the ambulance entrance, pushing a rolling stretcher. It was clear that some major emergency was taking place.

When the ambulance backed up to the E.R., the medical team opened the ambulance door. I peered in and saw an EMT doing CPR compression on a young man, Jeffrey, while the medical team unloaded him and wheeled him immediately into the cardiac treatment area. As the paramedic gave his report to the attending physician, the assisting doctors and nurses were busy with their assigned tasks. A doctor saw me standing idle and said, "Stand on the step stool and keep the chest compressions going."

I did as I was told and I had a chance to see the patient up close. I'd never seen such a well-developed and handsome young man before. He seemed like the essence of a Greek god, like an ancient statue in a museum. Jeffrey was an eighteen-year-old college freshman. He had been a straight A-student in high school and an All State athlete. In his freshman year in college, he made the dean's honor list and won a spot on the varsity baseball team. His future looked very bright.

That afternoon during a baseball game Jeffery had collapsed while running toward first base. An ambulance and crew were on hand and instantly EMTs began evaluating Jeffrey and found he was in cardiac arrest. Emergency cardiac resuscitation efforts were begun and Jeffrey was loaded into the ambulance. He arrived at the E.R. less than ten minutes later.

The medical team worked on Jeffrey for what seemed an eon but was probably about thirty minutes. They tried every known medical intervention but they just couldn't get his heart started again. Finally, the attending physician told the team to stop. Jeffrey was dead.

At that moment, something extremely unusual happened in the E.R. Everyone in the cardiac treatment area, including myself, started crying. That was unusual because medical personnel frequently see people die and they become immune to it to a certain extent. But each of us saw in Jeffrey's death the loss of his life's expectations just as his adult life was beginning. And each of us reacted to that tragedy by relating it to either our own children or some other young person we knew. It was the premature loss of everything Jeffrey had to look forward to that moved everyone so deeply.

A diagnosis of a chronic illness can feel similar to premature death because it means the loss of or decrease in your expectations for the future. It is as if you're driving down a country road on a sunny day and as you come around a sharp curve, the road suddenly comes to an end and there is an eclipse of the sun. You are enveloped in darkness with nowhere to go. In this chapter we will look at ways to counteract that terrible feeling of darkness.

Mind Struggles: Pessimism versus Optimism

Chronic illness can create a perception that your future is bleak and that your expectations have been greatly diminished or destroyed. This mindset can let loose very damaging negative emotions such as grief and despair and induce a high level of damaging stress. This is an intense mental crisis that will trigger a fight-or-flight reaction, a condition discussed earlier in this book. At this point the mind has to choose between two alternative views of your future: pessimistic and optimistic. A decision in favor of pessimism will cause you to retreat from your future. You mentally raise your hands in surrender, stop fighting your illness, and allow negative emotions to overwhelm you. A decision in favor of optimism will punch through the dark cloud of pessimism so that you can see a brighter future ahead of you.

It is human nature to become emotional about the future when bad things happen to you. In difficult situations, an emotional response often creates a pessimistic attitude. So how can you help yourself to reject pessimism and choose to see an optimistic future even when things are quite difficult? I suggest using the approach used by medical personnel to evaluate a medical emergency. Ask and answer these questions for yourself:

What has happened?

Is this a life-threatening situation? (Are you about to die?)

What needs to be done to prevent further injury?

What are the immediate treatment options?

When you ask yourself these or similar questions, your mental processes will automatically shift from the emotional portion of your brain (the limbic system) to the thinking area (the neocortex). As you begin thinking about your situation, your view of it will change as you start to consider alternative courses of action. Optimism can begin to displace pessimism and a new and brighter perspective of your future life begins to take shape.

Optimism Is a Human Trait

Until recently, optimism and pessimism were thought to be traits associated with specific personality types such as extrovert and introvert. Since the mid-1990s, neuroscientists, psychologists, and researchers in related fields have discovered that optimism is an inherited factor characteristic of all humans. Furthermore, they have located specific areas of the brain that are involved in producing an optimistic attitude.

When the uniquely human neurological functions of optimism and visualization (the ability to imagine a situation at another moment in time) are combined, it is possible to project a positive outcome for future activity. In fact, it has been established that people tend to be overly optimistic in estimating how things will turn out in the future. This extra-positive view of the future, known as the "optimism bias," serves a very important purpose in human activities. It propels people to take action because of a belief that their actions will lead to good results.

Pessimism, on the other hand, is most often the result of imposed values and attitudes or negative personal experiences. Parents, teachers, relatives, and other people you have frequent social contact with are the most common sources of imposed values. They are most likely to tell you what they think is the "right" profession, "correct" marriage partner, the "only" religion, or "appropriate" social behavior.

"You can do better than that."

"My parents always said that I was the dumbest kid in the family and I wouldn't amount to anything in life."

Pessimism about the future can also result from previous negative experiences. I have a friend, Philip, who wanted to become a doctor as long as he could remember. Upon graduation from college, he was accepted at an outstanding medical school in Europe, so clearly he was a talented scholar. However, he failed the comprehensive exam at the end of his first year because he wasn't used to the European system of yearly rather than progressive exams. He was not allowed to repeat the first year or to continue in the program. His friends encouraged him to apply to other medical schools, but he refused to because he was pessimistic about his chances of acceptance.

All professional activities that involve performance—such as acting, dance, music, and athletics—are subject to the possibility of rejection. After receiving several rejections, the performer may become pessimistic about future opportunities to perform and stop trying to win new opportunities. The same can happen to a patient who has several negative medical experiences. That is unfortunate because <u>a successful outcome may be directly related to the number of attempts you and your doctors make to solve your medical problems</u>.

Positive Psychology Can Help You Change Your Perspective

Positive psychology is a new branch of psychology initiated by Dr. Martin Seligman in 1998, when he was president-elect of the American Psychological Association. The purpose of this new scientific field of research is to examine the experiences and the personal, institutional, and cultural qualities that can assist anyone to achieve a life worth living.

In an article introducing the new approach, Dr. Seligman and his colleague, Mihaly Csikszentmihalyi, wrote:

> *Psychology is not just the study of pathology, weakness, and damage; it is also the study of strength and virtue. Treatment is not just fixing what is broken; it is nurturing what is best. Psychology is not just a branch of medicine concerned with illness or health; it is much larger. It is about work, education, insight, love, growth.*

[T]he disease model does not move psychology closer to the prevention of . . . problems. Indeed, the major strides in prevention have come largely from a perspective focused on systematically building competency, not on correcting weakness.

Prevention researchers have discovered that there are human strengths that act as buffers against mental illness: courage, future mindedness, optimism, interpersonal skill, faith, work ethic, hope, honesty, perseverance, and the capacity for flow and insight, to name several.

The major psychological theories have changed to undergird a new science of strength and resilience . . . [I]ndividuals are now seen as decision makers, with choices, preferences, and the possibility of becoming masterful, efficacious, or in malignant circumstances, helpless and hopeless.

This science and practice will also reorient psychology back to its two neglected missions — making normal people stronger and more productive and making high human potential actual.[4]

This new branch of psychology has important implications for you and all chronically ill patients. The comments quoted above mean that you already possess personal strengths that you can use to overcome the limitations of your illness in order to achieve a meaningful and fulfilling life. Furthermore, your strengths can be used to overcome weaknesses in your personality.

One of the first goals of Dr. Seligman and other positive psychologists was to search for, identify, and classify positive human characteristics. In the few years since the announcement of this new psychological field this goal has been achieved. The team examined the teachings of major philosophies and religions extending thousands of years back, including Aristotle, Plato, Buddha, and many more important contributors to the understanding of human nature and thought from both Eastern and Western civilizations.

They found that there are six virtues that are common to nearly every one of the traditions they examined. Furthermore, their research revealed that twenty-four specific human types of strength, which they called Values in Action, can be used by anyone to develop the six virtues. The six virtues and their related Values in Action, taken from Jessica Coleman's book *Optimal Functioning: A Positive Psychology Handbook*, are shown below.[5]

1. **Strength of Wisdom and Knowledge**
   - Creativity
   - Curiosity
   - Open-mindedness
   - Love of Learning
   - Perspective

2. **Strength of Courage**
   - Bravery
   - Persistence
   - Integrity
   - Vitality

3. **Strength of Humanity**
   - Love
   - Kindness
   - Social Intelligence

4. **Strength of Justice**
   - Citizenship
   - Fairness
   - Leadership

5. **Strength of Temperance**
   - Forgiveness and Mercy
   - Humility
   - Prudence
   - Self-Regulation

6. **Strength of Transcendence**
   - Appreciation of Beauty and Excellence
   - Gratitude
   - Hope
   - Humor
   - Spirituality

As you study the above list, you will see that the full life it describes goes far beyond the limitations imposed by a chronic illness. These values and traits help you realize that your illness is only one aspect of your life, not your whole life. Your illness no doubt leaves room for you to incorporate many of the above qualities into your life.

All this may sound wonderful and uplifting when presented in the halls of academia. But can it be applied in a practical way that you can use? The answer is yes. The following suggestions contained in Jessica Colman's book may help you to use positive psychology to move beyond the boundaries of your disease.

1. Start with a strength assessment. Use the list of Values in Action to evaluate your strengths and weaknesses.

2. Set goals based on your strengths. This is a critical step. You need to know where you want to go before taking any actions.

3. Use strengths to manage weaknesses. Using positive psychology is like riding a bicycle: to keep going you need to stay in balance and use your strengths to offset your weaknesses.

4. Keep an eye out for strengths in yourself and others. Keep growing! Looking for and finding strengths in others will provide you with insight as to how other people are using their strengths. As you develop a sensitivity for seeing strengths in other people, you may find or unlock strengths in yourself that you were not aware of.

Create a New Perspective

If you believe in your self-worth and are willing to work your way forward, one step at a time, toward a better future, you can achieve it. Don't allow yourself to fall into negativity or self-pity. You can create a new and positive perspective for your future life using the following four steps:

1. Put yourself in a positive environment. Keep your home and workplace brightly lit. "Think Green" and use compact fluorescent lightbulbs that emit more light while using less energy. I am continually amazed to find people who express misgivings about their future living in poorly lit homes. As soon as they use brighter lights, their outlooks also brighten.

Surround yourself with positive-thinking people who see the world as a "glass half full." There is nothing more discouraging than the negative comments of a dour person whose only objective is to make you equally negative. Happy people attract other happy people.

Participate in organizations that support your positive qualities. Community is important because members can be supportive of your efforts and offer helpful suggestions and insights you might not have thought of. Most importantly, you are not alone your endeavors.

2. Feed your optimism by identifying and developing your personal strengths. Make a list of your positive qualities and checkmark the strongest ones. Rate them on a scale from 1 (slightly strong) to 5 (very strong). You can use your strongest qualities to offset the weaker ones. If you need some assistance in identifying your positive qualities, take a look at the twenty-four values presented in the positive psychology handbook mentioned above.

3. Visualize a new perspective for yourself and your life.
Visualization involves forming strong mental images of things
you want, so that they become installed in your mind and
you're more likely to take action to make them happen. Find a
peaceful place where you can be alone. I like to listen to Gregorian chants or choral music when I am visualizing. Make
yourself comfortable, close your eyes, and imagine who you
want to be in the future and how you want to live your life.
Begin with the broadest aspects and get a general idea of the
new things you want to do. Then fill in the details as they
become clearer to you. Come back to your sanctuary often to
continue constructing your new perspective. Don't be afraid
to change one or all aspects. Play with your vision until you're
satisfied with it.

4. Live your new perspective. Implement your vision for
your life a little at a time until you are comfortable with your
new perspective and your new life experiences.

Ein-shei Chen's Story

Ein-shei Chen and her husband, Jin-lai Chang, immigrated to the United States from Taiwan. By all measures of
life, they have made positive contributions to America's social
fabric. Living in southern California, he established a successful orthodontic practice, she became a certified practitioner of
traditional Chinese medicine (acupuncture), and together they
raised two sons and a daughter. Any description of Ein-shei
would have to include the words *intelligent, active, engaged,*

and *involved*. In her own words, this is what she was doing before she became ill.

> I was teaching at the university of South Bay in California. Before I developed ALS, I was a certified practitioner of traditional Chinese medicine as well. When I was a student, I was the chairperson of the Student Union. I was chosen to be the chairperson of the alumni association after graduation as well, and I was active to promote exchange of Chinese medicine academics between China and America. In addition to that, I took in part of local activities in South California and was also a very active member of the Women's Club in Garden Grove City, Chinese Lions Club in Orange County, Taiwan Hometown Association and Overseas Chinese Commerce Association in South California.[6]

Her daughter says that list leaves out a number of other organizations.

In 1995, Ein-shei was diagnosed with Amyotrophic lateral sclerosis (ALS), also referred to as Lou Gehrig's disease in the United States and Motor Neurone Disease in Great Britain and other nations. ALS is a degenerative disease of the central nervous system that attacks the nerves that control motion and coordination, especially the muscles of the neck, arms, hands, legs, and feet. Over time, it becomes increasingly difficult for the person to stand, walk, speak, swallow, or use the hands. However, the disease does not affect the five senses or the ability to think.

Ein-shei's doctor told her that she had about two years to live. She reacted as would any other patient to such a devastating diagnosis. She retreated into herself, became depressed, and refused to even allow her friends to visit her. One of her greatest concerns about the disease was the prospect of undergoing a bronchotomy (also called tracheotomy or laryngotomy—an incision into the airway when respiration becomes compromised), something she did not want to have. At the time, her oldest son was attending the University of California at Berkeley. He became so concerned that he transferred to the University of California at Los Angeles (UCLA) to be near her. Upon graduation from UCLA, he spent two years as her caregiver before entering medical school.

Following her diagnosis, Ein-shei attended the monthly meetings of the local ALS support group. It was there that she met a patient who had already survived twenty years with ALS and did not require a bronchotomy. It was then that she "gained courage to live with ALS."

Ein-shei and her husband returned to Taiwan when her condition became severe, because she has an extensive family support structure there, which helped her regain her positive outlook on life. She described her daily life with ALS:

Today, I have two caregivers, one from the Philippines and the other from Indonesia. They take care of me in turn, and exchange their shift once a week. I miraculously have been enjoying my life more than 13 years since my diagnosis. My success is accomplished with a comfortable environment for home care, and the support of my family (parents, sisters and brothers, relatives, friends, husband and sons and daughter), as well as my own optimistic nature and my attitude respecting life. Today, I spend my regular daily life, without having bronchotomy as well. I have three meals a day as healthy people do. Only difference is that I need longer time to eat with the help of a caregiver.[7]

If you read Ein-shei's case history and watch her video[8] you will learn that she spends a considerable amount of time each day communicating by e-mail and webcam with other ALS patients, her family, and friends. I received an e-mail from her that contained five short sentences. Her daughter told me that the e-mail probably took her twenty minutes to construct. To type an e-mail, Ein-shei uses her left large toe (the only muscle she can control) to press a switch button that activates a special computer program, causing a cursor to scroll through an on-screen alphabet. When the cursor reaches the letter she wants, she presses the button to enter the letter into her message. The special software allows her to use all the e-mail features through the toe button. But as you can imagine, it takes a long time to write one brief e-mail.

Ein-shei also visits patients accompanied by her two aides, and often a family member. She says she hears amazing stories from the patients. She talks to them through an aide using an eye-gaze communication board. This device is commonly a large transparent sheet of plastic with the alphabet printed in large letters or groups of letters on one side. Ein-shei looks at the board and blinks when she is looking at a letter or group she wants. The aide calls out the letter or group of letters to confirm Ein-shei's choice. This is repeated until Ein-shei is finished constructing a word, phrase, or sentence. Then the aide reads out loud what Ein-shei has "said" with her eyes.

Ein-shei has not allowed her disease to keep her from achieving goals she had set for herself, especially ALS activities and projects. She has traveled to fifteen countries to attend and speak at ALS conferences. She is the current president of the Motor Neurone Disease Association of Taiwan.

Ein-shei is not a person who takes "no" for an answer. Her daughter recounts that some relatives in Taiwan did not want to take her to a wedding and gave various reasons for not including her. She attended. In November 2011, the government of Taiwan opened an ALS health center with a capacity for thirty-five patients in Taipei, the capital. It is the first ALS clinic in Asia. Ein-shei lobbied hard for a similar facility for her city, Taichung. She won. The Taichung ALS health center opened in January 2012.

Despite all her ALS-related activities, family relations are at the core of Ein-shei's life perspective. She is in frequent contact with her children, who live in the United States. The oldest son is a surgeon, the daughter is a healthcare consultant, and the youngest just graduated from law school.

If you need any further encouragement to adopt a new and positive perspective on your life, I suggest you read Ein-shei's story and watch the video. You will be inspired by her desire to live a quality life and to assist other ALS patients.

I asked Ein-shei to answer three questions that only she could answer. Here are the insightful answers she sent me via e-mail.

1. What motivated you to change from being depressed about your illness to a positive state of mind?

In the beginning, I didn't like people knowing that I was sick because I had just gotten my acupuncture license and I was planning to open an acupuncture clinic at that time. I was too busy reviewing my books and studying to treat my own disease. So I decided that I was going to lie low for a while until I got my health back. I didn't want to see any friends who came to visit me (I don't think I was depressed then) because I thought I could cure it through Chinese medicine. But the fact was that I was getting worse. Finally I gave up the dream of opening a clinic. I did feel a little disappointed in myself. The love from my family did cheer me up, especially when my oldest son transferred from Berkeley to UCLA to be closer to home and to take care of me for two years before he went to medical school. Then I started to work on improving ALS patients' daily life.

2. You have traveled to at least fifteen countries to speak about ALS. What is the purpose of your extensive travels?

I did travel to more than fifteen countries. There were two main reasons for my extensive travels:

First, I knew that in the very near future I would be confined to my bed. I wanted to input as much beautiful scenery into my brain as I could so that I would have a lot beautiful memories to enjoy after I was confined to my bed.

Second, I wish I can convince all people who leave their ALS handicapped patients at home to bring them out to have more decent lives. (ALS patients are so quiet. Most patients have been treated like vegetables. It is very cruel to the patients. Their minds still work and it is like they are being put in a jail where they can't even move).

3. What do you want to say to ALS and other chronically ill patients? What is your message?

I have four things to tell other patients:

1. Be well-prepared for the coming situation. Understand your condition and make sure those around you understand how best to support you while you can still communicate effectively.

2. Master the computer. Today's technology will allow you to communicate with the world, even if the only thing you can move is a big toe or an eyelid—but you have to know how to navigate the computer.

3. Design your daily life in a way that fits you and is easy to maintain. This is a part of being prepared. Make sure you have a simple routine that is easy for caretakers to follow and that they know will satisfy you. Nothing is harder on your caretakers than trying to guess what it is that you want, and failing.

4. Don't be afraid to ask for help. Our pride and dignity will initially get in the way of asking for help. Learning to understand that people really do want to help, and that their sympathy and goodwill is well intentioned, will help pave the way for a better life.

When I am happy, people around me are happy. So it is very important not to be afraid to ask for help and make yourself comfortable. Then you can be happy. Everybody can be happy.

Optimism is natural to humans, but you need to give optimism a chance to flourish. If you can't talk yourself into a new perspective, ask yourself, "What would I do today if I weren't feeling miserable?" Then just get up and go do it. Put yourself in an environment that feels uplifting. Associate with people who are living the way you want to live, doing the things you want to do. If you do those things long enough, even against your will, you will feel things start to change inside yourself and you will be more willing to visualize a new future for yourself, constructed around your strengths and abilities. Finally, learn about how people like Ein-shei Chen adapt to their situations and develop a new perspective to find new opportunities and live meaningfully even with a serious chronic illness.

CHAPTER 7

Be Inspired by Others
to Overcome Adversity

This is the greatest lesson a child can learn. It is the greatest lesson anyone can learn. It has been the greatest lesson I have learned: If you persevere, stick with it, work at it, you have a real opportunity to achieve something. Sure, there will be storms along the way. And you will not reach your goal right away. But if you do your best and keep a true compass, you'll get there.
—Ted Kennedy, *True Compass: A Memoir*

THE HUMAN ORGANISM—BODY, MIND, AND SPIRIT—is like a car. If you park your car in the driveway with the engine idling, it's not going to go anywhere. It just sits there wasting gas. It's possible for the body to stay alive in idle mode, as when a comatose patient is kept alive by artificial means. But that's not really living, is it? <u>To be alive you need to be going somewhere—making plans, setting goals, pursuing aspirations</u>. This is what we humans were designed for.

Your initial impulse when you first learned you had a serious chronic illness may have been to list all the things you would no longer be able to do. That's a normal response. But in this chapter I hope to show you that you can shift your focus away from what you *can't* do to what you *can* do. When you do that, small miracles may start to occur, as you will see in this chapter.

Our spirit is never satisfied when we are operating in idle mode. Despair is a dark force that lowers our operating speed down to idling. *Hope* is the spark plug that ignites the force we call living.

My purpose in this chapter is to ignite your hope and determination no matter what hurdles your illness has placed in your way. You are going to meet three chronically ill people who achieved their seemingly impossible goals through the forces of hope and character. Very few of my readers will have experienced the profound state of disability that Mark O'Brien and Stephen Hawking lived with for most of their lives. Perhaps you will be able to identify with Ted Kennedy's illness. All of their stories are about transcending the apparent limitations of illness and going beyond what was expected of them.

I am sharing these stories with you so that you will realize how connected you are to others who have also experienced a debilitating illness, and see greater possibilities for yourself. The constant companion of chronic illness is loneliness. Depression and despair can rob you of your desire to be with people and make you withdraw into solitude. You need to do the opposite of what your feelings are telling you to do, and seek fellowship with other people in order to be inspired by their life stories.

It is a condition of life that virtually everyone, no matter what socioeconomic class they belong to, will experience a devastating event at one time or another. If you read the tabloids you realize that the rich and famous have their equal share of troubles. It may be the death of a loved one, a failed marriage, an overwhelming financial problem, a family member who develops an addiction, sudden unemployment—the list goes on and on. Each of these life events can cause the same withdrawal response as a devastating chronic illness diagnosis—at a time when we most need the comfort and support of others.

Now I invite you into the intimate lives of three people whose stories will no doubt inspire you to continue your life with courage, imagination, and hope.

Mark O'Brien: The Mind Is Greater than the Body

Mark O'Brien was a young man who insisted on taking his full place in society as a student, journalist, and poet in spite of a medical condition that would have been totally disabling to a less determined person.

Mark was born in Boston in 1949 and grew up in Sacramento, California. At the age of six he contracted polio, a disease caused by a virus that attacks the nerve fibers that control muscle activity and can cause complete paralysis within several hours. There was and still is no cure for polio. Polio affected all of Mark's muscles below the neck, including those that control breathing. In those days, polio victims who were unable to breathe on their own were placed in a heavy, bulky, noisy iron lung that enclosed the body from the neck downward. It weighed an incredible nine hundred pounds and was very difficult to move around. Once placed in an iron lung, patients were imprisoned in the device for the rest of their life.

Mark O'Brien gradually became totally dependent on the iron lung to keep him alive.

Most polio patients in the 1950s were cared for in nursing homes. Mark's parents, however, chose to care for him at home. It was an effort of great dedication on their part to take care of him and ensure the proper operation of the iron lung twenty-four hours a day, every day.

In 1978, at the age of twenty-nine, Mark was accepted as a freshman at the University of California at Berkeley, where he majored in English literature. He and his iron lung moved to a small apartment in Berkeley. With the help of healthcare attendants, notetakers, and a new organization called the Center for Independent Living, he lived in his apartment and commuted to classes on a motorized gurney that carried him in his iron lung.

As an English literature major Mark had to write a lot of papers. He initially dictated his papers to assistants who typed them for him. Later he learned to use a mouth stick to strike the keys of a typewriter, one letter at a time. When word processors became available, he used the same technique to type his assignments electronically.

In his sophomore year, Mark published an essay about independent living, launching his career in journalism. He graduated from college at age thirty-three and decided to go to graduate school. He applied to the University of California's Graduate School of Journalism and was rejected several times. He ultimately prevailed when the school finally agreed to accept a severely handicapped student. By this time, his health had deteriorated further and he wasn't able to undertake his graduate studies — but he opened the door for other disabled students to be admitted to graduate schools.

Mark's journalism career included working throughout his life as an editor for Pacific News Service. He was also a freelance writer and his articles appeared in the San Francisco *Chronicle* and the *Examiner*, as well as the *National Catholic Reporter*. Although his ability to travel and conduct interviews was limited, the highlight of his career was an interview of physicist Stephen Hawking.

Mark wrote three volumes of poems: *Breathing, The Man in the Iron Lung*, and *Love and Baseball*. In 1997 film maker Jessica Yu won an Academy Award for her documentary about Mark's life and work, *Breathing Lessons: The Life and Work of Mark O'Brien*.

Mark died in 1999 at age fifty. The development of the polio vaccine by Dr. Jonas Salk came a year too late for Mark. In 1955 there were nearly twenty-nine thousand cases of polio in the United States. Two years later, the number of cases fell to six thousand. At the time of Mark's death, polio had been eliminated in the United States and there were only slightly more than one hundred patients still living in an iron lung.

If Mark O'Brien had not contracted polio, he would probably have lived a normal middle-class American life. He would have played sports, continued his education through graduate school, married, and had a family. He would have held a regular job, traveled, and pursued his broad interests. Once he was confined to an iron lung, he was cut off from all of those activities. For the average polio patient, the one and only challenge was to simply stay alive; to keep breathing. Most patients relegated to care in a nursing home did not fare well and experienced shortened life expectancies.

Mark set a challenge for himself: to live as normal a life as possible within the constraints of his iron lung. He succeeded beyond anyone's expectations because of the excellent care and encouragement he receive from his parents, the support of many individuals and organizations who believed in his potential, and, most importantly, his personal qualities. Once he set a goal for himself, he never gave up. He persisted against all odds and went far beyond reasonable expectations of a person living in an iron lung.

Mark's goal was to become a working journalist. During his nineteen-year career he continually developed his skills as an editor, essayist, and poet. All this was achieved using a mouth stick to tap out one letter at a time on a word processor while trapped in an infernal giant bellows that noisily forced air in and out of his lungs! His wit, sarcasm, and desire to be normal are given expression in Jessica Yu's documentary.

Mark's poem "Breathing" conveys his determination to hold onto his connection to life:

> Grasping for straws is easier;
> You can see the straws.
> "This most excellent canopy, the air, look you,"
> Presses down upon me
> At fifteen pounds per square inch,
> A dense, heavy, blue-glowing ocean,
> Supporting the weight of condors
> That swim its churning currents.
> All I get is a thin stream of it,

A finger's width of the rope that ties me to life
As I labor like a stevedore to keep the connection.

Mark's legacy is the philosophy that guided his life and inspired all who came in contact with him: "The mind is greater than the body." His legacy is a challenge to every chronically ill person. How persistent are you, and how much effort and hardship are you willing to endure to achieve your goal?

Stephen Hawking: Following Passion Beyond All Obstacles

Stephen Hawking is one of the world's best known and most accomplished theoretical physicists. Perhaps Einstein's name is more recognized worldwide, but Hawking's work actually goes beyond the groundwork laid by Einstein. It also extends far beyond the academic world: hundreds of thousands of laypeople around the world are familiar with his work through his best-selling popular science books, including *A Brief History of Time*, that excited interest in cosmology (the study of the nature and origin of the universe).

Stephen Hawking has been honored throughout his prolific forty-year career with some of the most prestigious positions and awards bestowed by the scientific community. He achieved that status despite the almost impossible burden of ALS—the same illness that struck Ein-shei Chen (chapter 6).

Stephen Hawking was diagnosed with ALS at age twenty-one while a graduate student at Cambridge University. At that time (the early 1950s) the survival time for ALS sufferers was thought to be three to five years. At his website Hawking describes his initial reaction of shock and confusion when he learned he had ALS:

> The realization that I had an incurable disease, that was likely to kill me in a few years, was a bit of a shock. How could something like that happen to me? Why should I be cut off like this? . . . Not knowing what was going to happen to me, or how rapidly the disease would progress, I was at a loose end. The doctors told me to go back to Cambridge and carry on with the research I had just started in general relativity and cosmology. But I was not making much progress because I didn't have much mathematical background. And, anyhow, I might not live long enough to finish my Ph.D.[9]

Hawking's challenge at that point was twofold. First he needed to move through the S.A.R.A. stages of grieving to an acceptance of his disease. Then he needed to establish a goal that he could achieve despite the continuing progress of his disease.

Hawking's biggest academic problem during his undergraduate years at Oxford University was boredom. His very bright mind did not find much challenge in the courses he needed to complete for his degree. When he found a field of study that lit his passion — theoretical physics — he took off like a rocket, barely slowed in his career or his personal life by his recent diagnosis. He won a prestigious research fellowship, completed his PhD early, married, and had children.

All the while, ALS was continuing to weaken Hawking's body. By the time he received his PhD he was using a wheelchair to move about. His speech had deteriorated so much that only people who knew him well could understand what he was saying. His work continued, however, and he quickly became a leading authority in theoretical physics. In 1972 he was elected to membership in the Royal Society as one of its youngest members. That same year, he received the Albert Einstein Award, considered to be the highest award in the field of theoretical physics. All this by the age of thirty, with an illness that was supposed to have killed him in five years!

In 1979 Hawking was elected to a prestigious mathematics position at Cambridge. He retired from that chair thirty years later, at age sixty-seven. During those three decades, he established a reputation as a leading expert on black holes and the origin of the universe. Although his mathematical conception of the universe is understood by only a very small group of skilled mathematicians, he has been able to communicate his thinking in ways that can be understood and appreciated by the general public. He is still working and it is probably too soon to predict what his final legacy will be.

As of this writing, Hawking is virtually paralyzed throughout his body. He is totally dependent on his team of healthcare aides and assistants to sustain his life functions and to continue working. To type on his specialized computer, he uses his cheek—one of the few muscles in his body that still functions. His lifetime achievements would be amazing if he had been in good health. How could a person with such limited physical functioning reach such heights of accomplishment and become known around the world?

Fortunately for Hawking, as his ALS progressed, how society perceived the potential of people with disabilities was evolving, leading to greater efforts to support them in all areas of their lives. Hawking has had support from a virtual army of people who meet his daily physical requirements and assist him with his professional endeavors, enabling him to write articles and books, deliver lectures, and give interviews.

Great strides have been made with assistive technology for people with disabilities. By sheer good timing, as Hawking's physical capabilities declined, the first personal computer was developed. Advances in hardware, software, and other equipment facilitated his needs for communication and mobility: a personal computer mounted on the arm of his wheelchair; a speech synthesizer that allows him to create lectures and respond to questions; a telephone device; remote controls for ordinary home electronic devices and for opening doors and turning on lights, and so on.

Most importantly, Stephen Hawking is driven by a ceaseless curiosity about the physical sciences, an indomitable spirit, and determination to pursue his goals as long as he can continue to express what his mind is thinking. "My goal is simple," he said. "It is complete understanding of the universe, why it is as it is and why it exists at all."[10] That internal drive fueled Hawking's tremendous productivity, leading to publication of his best-selling books, considerable income, and widespread attention from people and organizations that wanted to support him. In a word, Hawking followed his passion beyond all obstacles in his path, and millions of people and great resources were drawn to him.

Stephen Hawking's story gives hope to all chronically ill patients. His life's work says, If you can think and reason, you are alive and can still be an active member of the human family.

Edward Kennedy: Rising Above Personal Failure to Extraordinary Public Service

Seventy-eight-year-old Senator Edward Kennedy suffered a seizure at his Cape Cod home on May 20, 2008. He was taken to Massachusetts General Hospital, where doctors found that he had a very aggressive brain tumor. Patients with this type of brain cancer rarely live more than two years following the diagnosis. Kennedy lived fifteen months.

Senator Kennedy quickly sized up his medical prognosis and took stock of how he wanted to spend the remainder of his life. He decided that he was not done working on the political and social issues that had been at the heart of his forty-seven-year career. He set two goals that he wanted to achieve before he died: to see Barack Obama elected as the next president of the United States, and for Congress to enact a national healthcare bill. Kennedy saw in Barack Obama the liberal idealism that his brother Jack brought to the presidency. National healthcare reform had been an unfulfilled goal of the Democrats since the presidency of Harry Truman in the 1940s and a personal goal of Ted Kennedy since 1970, when he introduced a bill to provide national health insurance. He believed that Barack Obama was the presidential candidate who would lead the nation in implementing his lifelong goal of healthcare for all Americans.

To understand what motivated Ted Kennedy in the last year of his life—why he chose to continue working for the American people instead of withdrawing into more personal pursuits—you have to understand where he came from and the threads of his life. He was born in 1932 into one of America's wealthiest and most politically powerful families. His father, Joseph Kennedy, was extremely successful in business due to his shrewd business acumen and ability to use political influence to his advantage. Joseph Kennedy had great ambitions for his sons. He used his wealth and political influence to back the election of Jack Kennedy to the presidency and then to have Robert installed as attorney general. Ted was elected to fill the seat left by his brother in the Senate in 1962.

Despite the Kennedy family's great wealth, political power, and influence in American society, it has been a family beset by tragedy. Ted's three older brothers were all killed before they reached middle age. Joe Jr. was killed in action during World War II. Jack was assassinated in Dallas in 1963. The following year Robert was assassinated in Los Angeles while campaigning for president. Ted's oldest sister, Rosemary, had some type of intellectual challenge that was poorly understood in the early 1900s. Her condition worsened after a lobotomy and she was institutionalized. Kathleen, Ted's second oldest sister, died at twenty-seven in a plane crash.

Ted Kennedy's own life was marred by serious problems— many brought on by his own behavior—that almost ended his political career more than once. It took him many years to develop the maturity and good judgment he would need to become a leader in the Senate and champion of disadvantaged Americans. As an undergraduate at Harvard University, he was expelled for cheating on an examination, and only readmitted after serving in the army. In 1964 he was severely injured in a plane crash and spent months in recovery.

In 1969, after a party on Chappaquiddick Island, Massachusetts, Ted lost control of his car and drove off a bridge. His passenger, Mary Jo Kopechne, died and Ted's conduct after the accident would stain his political career for the rest of his life. The incident forced him out of his position as Senate Majority Whip and ended any thoughts he had of campaigning for president. However, he was reelected to the Senate in 1970 and gained the chairmanship of the Senate Health Committee.

Ted Kennedy reached the nadir of his political and personal life after an episode at the family compound in Miami Beach in 1991, when his nephew William Kennedy Smith was accused of raping a young woman. William was ultimately acquitted, but Ted's involvement in the incident resulted in the lowest poll ratings of his political career.

Each of these tragic events helped to shape Ted Kennedy's emergence as one of the most effective U.S. senators in history. He was able to turn adversity, misfortune, and personal error to his profit by learning from each incident and clarifying his goals. After the Chappaquiddick incident, maturity dominated his reckless nature. Within his first year as chair of the Senate Health Committee, he introduced a bill for national health insurance. Over the next thirty-nine years, he would become the champion of ordinary Americans and introduce bills on civil rights, immigration, education, and health. His legislative successes were often due to his ability to cross the aisle and work with Republicans to cosponsor bills. He worked with President Bush to gain passage of the No Child Left Behind Act. In this new phase of his life Ted found happiness in his personal life as well when he married his second wife, Victoria Reggie, in 1992.

Ted Kennedy's greatest social and political dream was healthcare for all Americans. When his son Ted. Jr. lost a leg to cancer at age twelve, Ted Sr. saw firsthand what families go through when a child has a major illness. In a speech on April 3, 2008, Kennedy described how that experience marked him:

> I knew my child was going to have the best possible care because I had the health insurance of the United States Senate. And I knew that no parent [in his son's research program] had the kind of coverage that I had. That kind of choice for any parent in this country is absolutely unacceptable and wrong, my friends.
>
> I can tell you this. When every member of the United States Senate comes into the Senate and signs in, they sign a little card in two places. One is for their salary and the other is for their health insurance. Now Senator Brown of Ohio, to his credit, will not accept it until the people of Ohio get it. Every other member of the U.S. Senate has accepted it. And for the fifteen times I have fought on the floor of the United States Senate, that we ought to have universal comprehensive coverage. And to listen to the voices on the other side [of the aisle] that have universal and comprehen-

sive coverage say, "No, it's the wrong time. We cannot afford it. It is the wrong bill at the wrong time."

My friends, if that health insurance is good enough for the members of the Congress of the United States, and good enough for the president of the United States, it is good enough for everybody in Montgomery county, good enough for everyone in Pennsylvania, and everybody across this country.[11]

Ted Kennedy knew that if a national healthcare bill was to be passed while he served in the Senate, he would need a Democratic president to be his partner in the effort. While he was under great pressure to support Hillary Clinton's bid for the presidency, he felt that her earlier failure to create an acceptable healthcare bill during Bill Clinton's presidency had strongly divided the nation. Therefore he decided to support Barack Obama's candidacy and to be influential in shaping Obama's healthcare platform. At the Democratic National Convention on August 26, 2008, he rose from his hospital bed, wracked with pain from kidney stones, and was brought to the convention hall to give his endorsement of Barack Obama. He rallied the delegates to his life's cause in his speech when he said, "And this is the cause of my life: new hope that we will break the old gridlock and guarantee that every American—north, south, east, west, young, old—will have decent, quality healthcare as a fundamental right and not a privilege."[12]

Ted's endorsement was the lift the Obama campaign needed to defeat Hillary Clinton. In accepting Kennedy's support, Obama essentially made a public vow to continue

Kennedy's work to pass a healthcare bill.

Despite his illness, Ted continued to work part-time on Senate matters. On July 9, 2009, six weeks before he died, he returned to the Senate to cast a crucial vote that defeated a Republican bill that would have reduced Medicare reimbursements to doctors. As the most powerful member of the Senate, he used his remaining time and energy to keep his colleagues focused on the issue of national healthcare reform at a time when the war in Iraq was dominating the headlines.

Ted Kennedy did not live to see a national healthcare bill enacted into the law of the nation. He died on August 25, 2009 — seven months before President Obama signed into law the legislation that Ted Kennedy spent his life working for, the Patient Protection and Affordable Care Act. The passage of that law reflects a monumental shift in our country's view of our duty to care for all of our citizens. Ted Kennedy's role in that shift cannot be overestimated. He remained at the forefront of our social consciousness for almost half a century.

What Will YOUR Legacy Be?

Mark O'Brien, Stephen Hawking, and Ted Kennedy have very different life stories. Their challenges, how they overcame them, their skills and resources, their life course, and their legacies are all unique. Yet there are many common threads in their stories: hope; overcoming terrible adversity; the determination to leave their mark on the world; focusing on the abilities and resources they had, rather than what they didn't have; the will to live the largest possible life beyond the limitations of their illness. Each of these individuals achieved much more than would have been expected of most people in their situation. When they encountered an obstacle that would have stopped anyone else in their tracks, they found ingenious ways of moving around and beyond those obstacles.

In each of these stories, you can see that the individuals separated themselves from their illness, realizing that if their body was no longer fully functioning as they hoped, they still had their mind and their spirit. They did not allow themselves to be defined by their illness, but by their passions and aspirations. They shifted their focus from their limitations to giving as much as they could to the world through the arts, science, politics, and sharing their wisdom in ways that touched ordinary people.

Lacking the full cooperation of their body, they rose to the occasion and applied the full strength of their *character*. Even with all of Ted Kennedy's inherited family wealth and power, in the end what allowed him to rise above his personal tragedies and failures and have a successful outcome and legacy was his character. "Character" here means acceptance of adversity, determination, and commitment to life no matter what your personal circumstances. At certain moments, Mark O'Brien, Stephen Hawking, and Ted Kennedy may have felt they had almost nothing on their side and that all was lost. They made sure that that stage of loss of hope was only temporary, and they set about moving far, far beyond that moment.

Because of how they chose to live their lives, each person I have written about left a legacy that far transcended their individual lives. The outcome of Ted Kennedy's work, for example, will continue to be significant over the next decade and beyond as our country transforms our healthcare system.

If you are tempted to say, "But I'm not Ted Kennedy! I don't have his wealth and power! I'm not great!" I invite you to reflect more deeply on the meaning and importance of your life. Around the world, millions of people are at this very moment overcoming unbelievable obstacles to live better lives. They are *ordinary people using extraordinary means* — determination, imagination, courage, and hard work — to move beyond their challenges and do extraordinary things. You can be great in your own life, in your own inspired way, by always seeking to expand your capabilities and what you give back to life. You can be great within your circle of family and your community.

The Jewish philosopher Martin Buber (1878–1965) believed that God speaks to us through the events of our lives, and that we answer God in the way we respond to those events. Let yourself be inspired by Mark O'Brien, Stephen Hawking, and Ted Kennedy: <u>think and act beyond your illness and press on with your life's purpose</u>. You will discover that each action you take will connect you more firmly with life and you will feel your hope rise with each step you take.

CHAPTER 8

Find Meaning in Your Life Story: A Life Worth Talking About

WHEN I ARRIVED AT THE hospice, a doctor approached and asked me to first visit the patient in room 19. He was dying and his family was with him. Over the years, I have been a witness to many different end-of-life situations, ranging from emotional outbursts of grief to the dark silence of family and friends patiently gathered around the patient in a dimly lit room. I did not expect the scene that met me when I entered this elderly gentleman's room.

Sunlight streamed through the windows overlooking the East River. Several family members were gathered around the man, conversing with each other. As I entered the room they stood up, smiled, and warmly welcomed me. The man's wife was the first to speak. She said, "Did you know that my husband was a World War II hero who saved his ship, the aircraft carrier Bunker Hill?" She described the actions he had taken in May 1945 to keep his ship afloat despite severe damage to the vessel and loss of over three hundred of the crew resulting from an attack by two kamikaze planes. She made sure that I wrote down the name of the book that told the story of the ship's survival and the crucial role her husband played. When she had finished telling her story, other family members cheerfully told me more stories about him that illustrated his character as a naval officer and his multiple careers in civilian life.

What was so unique and memorable about this end-of-life scene that I would want to share it with you? This man's family was celebrating his life by telling his life stories. Each family member had a different set of stories that recounted their own perspective and relationship to the man. Together, these stories created a picture that revealed the many dimensions of a man who had lived a life that impacted everyone who came within his sphere.

This man's name was Joseph P. Carmichael, Jr. Shortly after his death, the *New York Times* published an extensive obituary on October 1, 2011. It told how, as the ship's chief engineer, he kept the boilers — the heart of the ship — operating to provide water pressure for the fire hoses and power for vital equipment despite life-threatening conditions. Included with the article was a slide show of dramatic photographs of the burning vessel. Carmichael and the hundreds of men under his command fought against seemingly overwhelming odds. They won. They saved the ship and the lives of nearly three thousand sailors.

Joseph Carmichael's life story is truly awesome. Read his obituary and I expect that you too will be inspired. Knowing his life story is only possible for you and me because he told his stories to others, who repeated them to even more people.

Telling your life story is like dropping a pebble into a lake. The ripples caused by the impact of the stone on the water travel outward beyond your vision. Don't underrate the impact of your life story. Everyone's story is important.

Your Life Story Is Your Legacy

Everyone loves to hear a good story. Ever since the beginning of spoken language, before the invention of the printing press, personal and social histories were passed along from one generation to another by storytellers. If you've ever read a gripping autobiography, you know that people's personal stories can be fascinating and instructive. Did you ever wonder what would motivate a famous person to write down the intimate details of their past? I'm sure there are many reasons, but at the top of the list must be a need to be known as they really are, to set things straight, and to leave their story for posterity. These are needs that most people have.

Throughout this book I'm encouraging you, as a person with a chronic illness, to change the way that you think about yourself and your life, to better serve your goals. Organizing and telling your life story is an important part of thinking about your past, present, and future. Although your life has changed because of your illness, your past is not lost. In this chapter we will explore the many benefits of telling your life story, especially for people with a chronic illness, and the different ways you can go about it.

Your life story is your legacy. The ever-growing history of humankind is like a beautiful carpet, woven from thousands of individual yarns. Telling your life story will ensure that your "yarn" is included in the fabric of the history of humankind.

But your story is more than just a history. It contains hints from the past that are guideposts for finding meaning in life now and in the future.

How Telling Your Story Can Help You and Others

As a hospital chaplain I've listened to the life stories of dozens of ordinary people. I consider it an honor to be invited into someone's intimate world via their life story. I can assure you that everyone's story is interesting. You certainly don't need to be famous or highly accomplished in any special field to have an interesting story to tell. What is interesting is how your life is different from others': the challenges you encountered and how you overcame them; how you changed over your lifetime; the people, places, and things that you've loved; the contributions large and small that you've made. A life story doesn't need to be all rosy, either—people may be deeply touched by your saddest stories and find personal meaning in them.

Putting together your life story and sharing it with others is a sign that you are ready to deal with your illness in a positive and forceful way, that you have not given up the fight and have found the inner strength to continue living a meaningful life in spite of your health problems. That's a very positive message to send to others who are living with chronic illness.

People who know you, such as friends and family, may have come to see you in terms of the limitations imposed on you by your illness. Sharing the story of your past with them reminds them—and you—that you are more than a person with an illness. You are someone with an interesting past who is trying to live life to its fullest at the present time, and looking forward to the future. Seeing you in this light will come as a pleasant surprise to them.

A chronic illness often involves an endless stream of doctor visits, therapist sessions, lab tests, and a daily schedule of medicines. Your life seems bound by all these intrusions on your time. You may sometimes feel that you have been sent into a garden maze without a map. Or that you are merely a medical puppet and others are holding the strings that control your movements. This feeling of not being in control of your life can give rise to negative emotions, including depression, despair, and loss of hope and any meaning for your life. Most harmful to your well-being is the sense that you are alone; that no one else is experiencing or understands what you are going through.

Telling your life story can help you throw off these negative feelings by giving you a new, brighter perspective on your past, present, and future. Sharing your story with friends, family, and caregivers will be uplifting for them and enormously gratifying for you. Below are some of the benefits you will receive from telling your life story.

Find the meanings of your past. Whether you are eighteen or seventy-eight, your past life includes innumerable experiences: joys and sorrows, successes and failures, exciting adventures and your mundane daily life of work and family.

Those experiences paint a picture of a very special life: yours. Particularly meaningful are the lessons you have learned from your past experiences. They are signposts to the future for you and others who have had similar experiences.

New strength. You can be your own worst enemy when you see yourself as an incomplete, weak, or unfulfilled person because of your illness. When you take the time to consider your past, you will see that you have had many accomplishments, perhaps ones you haven't been aware of or didn't consider significant.

Seeing all that you've done in the past and all the hurdles you've overcome, you realize that you will be able to meet today's and tomorrow's challenges. Telling your life story will reveal the strengths that are propelling you positively into the future.

Pride. Sharing the story of your life with others generates a unique life force within you. Someone says, "I didn't know that you did that!" and you sit or stand a little taller, you straighten your shoulders, and a sly smile appears on your face as you recall your past accomplishments and adventures.

Finding purpose for your life. We all need to know that we have a reason for living and that we count for something in this world. If you have no purpose to your life, your energies are spent randomly, thrown here and there with no particular target in mind. In that case you are just biding your time, which is a painful way to finish out your life.

How can you find purpose for your life when a chronic illness has imposed limitations that you never expected? As you organize the pieces of your past life into a coherent story, a picture emerges of the values that have been important to you, reflecting who you really are beneath the veneer of your illness. Those are the values that you want to carry forward in the future. They may be expressed differently than in the past. If you can no longer ski black-diamond trails, perhaps you will find fulfillment as a ski instructor working with young people. If you love children and have already raised your own family, an elementary school would love to have you as a classroom grandparent.

When you focus on creating purpose for your life, your mental energy will intensify, and you will find that you can almost move mountains to achieve the goals you've committed yourself to. There is an adage, "If you don't know where you're going, anywhere will do." The counterpart of this old saying is, "If you know where you've been, you will know where you want to go next and how to get there." Telling your life story will help you understand where you've been.

Helping other patients. Your life story, how you have dealt with the challenges of your chronic illness, and what you are doing to go forward into the future are a vitally important story for others with the same illness. A recent medical study[13] demonstrated that listening to the stories of other patients with the same illness has as much benefit as taking medication, because it motivates people to adopt the same healthy behaviors as the storytellers. This astonishing finding demonstrates the well-known effectiveness of word-of-mouth communication.

Many people don't learn well from being taught by medical professionals who they don't know or trust, and who speak to them in medical jargon. Some patients are in denial and simply don't want to believe what their doctor tells them. Stories from other patients are different. These are ordinary people speaking in ordinary language about how their illness has affected them and how they are coping. Their story is believable, understandable, and personally meaningful. Their listeners can identify with them. That's why it's so important that you tell others the story of how you are coping with your illness. You can make a difference in the lives of other patients who need to hear your story. What you say can help them find the inner strength and direction that has been missing in their own lives.

Becoming a whole person rather than a faceless chart. Do you find that some of your healthcare providers think of you as just another patient, just another medical chart to process? They are undoubtedly very professional and courteous, but distant and impersonal. That does not have to be the case. By creating common points of interest through sharing your life story in medical settings, you can help medical personnel see you as a real and interesting person. Once your doctors know you better, the odds are very good that they will pay more attention to you, which translates into better healthcare.

Connecting with your support team. Just as you may be treated with indifference by healthcare providers, chronically ill patients often treat the members of their healthcare support team with the same indifference. Sharing your life story with your healthcare providers will help you reach out to them and see *them* as real people. That will make you more receptive to receiving care and following up on their recommendations.

Listening to Other People's Stories

Listening to or reading the life stories told by other people will be very helpful in preparing you to tell your own story. Patients—especially those with a chronic illness—frequently become so absorbed in their illness that that is all they talk about, over and over again. They lose sight of everything and everyone else around them. Listening to life stories told by others will help you to connect with other human beings, to look around you and notice all the interesting things that are happening in the world besides you and your illness.

To tell one's life story is a defining moment in anyone's life, but especially for a chronically ill patient. At this moment of truth, storytellers will share with you how they have struggled to deal with their life challenges and what meaning they have found in their lives. Most importantly, you can learn why they keep going, what goals they are striving to achieve.

These stories will stimulate your creativity by giving you ideas for what you want to include in your own life story. Once you start thinking about sharing your life story, you will realize that there is a great deal you could talk about.

For one of the best ways to enjoy other people's stories, see the section below on StoryCorps.

Finding Meaning in Your Past

You are a unique person. There has never been a person just like you in the history of humankind, with the same life story. Nor will there will ever be anyone exactly like you at any time in the future.

As you begin thinking about your past life, you will come to the recognition that you've come a long way. It has been a journey that no one could have predicted. You have not traveled over a straight and easy path. Instead, you have been on a winding road with twists and turns, ups and downs. You have endured storms and seen bright sunny days. Looking back, you may be amazed at how far you have come.

Looking back at your past is like climbing into the attic to see what is stored there. As you rummage around, you come across reminders of the challenges that you have met, endured, and conquered. As you did that, you grew as a person and took on many new skills and insights. These pearls of wisdom from your past need to be shared with other people.

Very few people have a smooth path through life — that's not what we're in this life for. Most of us take many years to learn important life lessons. Often our most instructive experiences are the hard ones, which can leave us feeling bewildered. We wonder, "Why did those things have to happen to *me*?" Telling your life story will help you make sense of the complex puzzle of all these events. As you piece your story together, look for the common threads that point to who you are and what's important to you. That will help you decide which elements you want to carry forward in your future.

But of course life is not all sorrows, either. The good parts of your life point also to the strengths in your character, how you have been appreciated by others, all that you have loved, what you've given to the world. Rejoice in those memories and share your joy with your listeners, readers, or viewers.

Choosing What to Tell

For some people, the biggest hurdle to telling their life story is deciding what to include from a long and rich life. The solution to that problem is very simple. Just choose one of the following options and get started. There is no required formula for telling your story. It's your story, so just tell it the way you want to. You can also switch from one method to another whenever you choose. Or you can mix and match as it suits you. The important thing is to get started.

1. *Begin with your earliest childhood memories*. This is the easiest and most common method people choose to get started. Start by giving the basic facts of your life: your name, when and where you were born, what kind of work you do or did, and where you currently live. Then provide the names of your father and mother, including their birthdates and birthplaces, occupations, and where they now live or date and place of death if deceased. Include the same type of information about your paternal and maternal grandparents. If anyone, including yourself, was born in another country, describe when, why, and how they came to this country. You may think that including this kind of information is not very important, but it is the foundation on which family histories are based. Family members and historians listening to your story years and decades from now will thank you for providing these essential facts.

2. *Selected periods of your life*. As with everyone, certain periods of your life stand out more in your memory. Begin with the stage of life that you want everyone to know about.

Why is it so memorable? Share your experiences; let the audience see things from your perspective.

3. Memorable experiences. Along the journey of your past life, there may have been some very special experiences that changed the course of your life or hold a very special meaning for you. It may have been an event that you witnessed or participated in. It may have historical significance or it may only be important to you, but it was very memorable. Perhaps it was someone special in your life who helped you along the way or gave you a new and better perspective on life.

A Good Place to Begin: StoryCorps

StoryCorps is a nonprofit organization created in 2003 to record the life stories of Americans of all backgrounds and beliefs. Since its establishment, StoryCorps has recorded more than 30,000 oral histories throughout the United States. It currently has recording facilities in New York, San Francisco, and Atlanta where participants can tell their stories. Each participant receives a free CD of the recorded story. Copies of all the stories are preserved in the American Folklife Center at the Library of Congress. Excerpts from StoryCorps interviews are presented on the National Public Radio weekly program, *Morning Edition.*

StoryCorps is a very good starting point for telling your life story. If you use a computer or have access to a computer at a library, use the search term storycorps.org to open the door to a vast storytelling resource. If you are not comfortable using a computer, the librarian can help you get started. Here are some of the helpful aids you will find at StoryCorps:

- You can listen to the life stories told by participants. Listening to their stories may give you ideas for what you want to say about your life.
- Some stories are so inspiring that StoryCorps has animated them and presents them on its website.
- Some of the stories are presented in two books and related CDs: *Mom: A Celebration of Mothers from StoryCorps*, which was a *New York Times* best seller, and *Listening Is an Act of Love*. Either of these books or CDs will provide you with an opportunity to read or hear the stories at your convenience.
- StoryCorps has created many different outreach initiatives to groups of people whose experiences are important to understanding what it means to be an American, including teachers, people with life-threatening illnesses, Latinos, African Americans, people with memory loss, those impacted by 9/11, and New Yorkers. You might want to participate in one of the initiatives.
- You can download a Do-It-Yourself instruction guide for recording your life story. This four-page guide includes everything you need to know about how to tell your story.

Different Ways to Tell Your Story

There are several different methods you can use to tell your story. The most common are listed below. Choose the one that is most familiar and comfortable for you, or try something new. There are advantages and disadvantages to each method.

Pen and paper. Today even many older people know how to use a computer, but some people still like to use pen and paper. This is the simplest and least expensive method. Unfortunately, many people who have grown up in the age of personal computers have handwriting that barely approaches legibility. The only real disadvantage of this method is that someone will have to transcribe your written notes to computerized text.

Typewriter. For several years after I began using a personal computer, I kept an IBM Selectric typewriter on a shelf to use when I had to complete a paper form or type a single label. If you choose to type your story, your sheath of typewritten pages will have to be converted to computer text if you want to preserve it electronically. However, this is very easily done by commonly available computer text-recognition software. You can get a friend to make the conversion for you or take it to any office equipment store that offers printing services, such as Fedex Kinkos. The computerized text will be saved in electronic form, most likely on a CD.

Computer. This is the easiest way to write your story, because it allows you to make changes at will by moving things around and adding and deleting parts. If you've never used a computer before, it might be worth your while to learn simple word-processing skills. Your local library may be able to provide you with a computer and instruction. You could also ask for a young person at a local school to help you—even an elementary student. When you print a copy of the computer text, be sure to print it on readily available acid-free paper. Paper produced by the cheaper acid method will disintegrate over time. Acid-free paper will last a very long time.

Tape recording. For most people, this is the method of choice. The equipment required is inexpensive, easily acquired, and simple to use. All you have to do is put a tape into the recorder, press the record button and start talking. (I prefer ninety-minute audio tapes, which provide forty-five minutes of recording on each side.) When you have filled a tape, be sure to protect your recording by pressing down on either of the plastic tabs on the top edge of the cassette. This prevents you from recording over previously recorded material. To reuse the cassette, just put some transparent tape over the opening.

The advantage of a tape-recorded story is that your listeners can hear your voice, creating a more direct personal connection with you. There are two disadvantages of a tape-recorded story. First, the tape will deteriorate over time. The lifespan of recording tape kept under household conditions is about fifteen years. To extend the life of the recorded material, it can be converted to a digitized computer text format or computerized text using voice-recognition software. However, all electronic media, such as audio tapes, video tapes, CDs and DVDs, have limited life spans. If you just want to tell your story in the easiest way, tape record it and let someone else worry about the complexities of electronic life spans.

If you will be tape recording your story, you will do yourself a big favor by using the StoryCorps Do-It-Yourself Instruction Guide. If you don't have a personal computer, ask your librarian to help you download a copy of this document from the StoryCorps website.

Video recording. A life story told in video form is a wonderful experience for the viewer. It captures all the nuances of the storyteller's personality and unspoken meanings associated with the story. However, it requires more complex recording equipment and someone competent in operating the video camera and sound recording. Video recordings — tape or computerized — have the same life span problems as other electronic media.

Photographs. Photos are an excellent way to tell your story, as they give the viewer an exact image of the important people and places in your life. To see an example of how photographs can be used to tell a history, look at any of the several hundred local history books published by Acadia Publishing. Your local bookstore or public library undoubtedly has several examples. All you need for your storytelling project are an album, the photographs you want to include, photo mounting materials available from any crafts store, and labels for captions for the photographs. A label-making machine can make it a lot easier to create captions. The disadvantage of a photo album is the limitation on how much text you can put on each label. However, you can overcome this by including written stories in your album, next to the photos. Photographs, especially black and white, have a very long life if protected from direct light in an album.

Artistic media. If you have a special talent in the arts, such as painting, drawing, or composing music, you might consider telling your life story creatively and artistically. Once you have created your work of art, it will be helpful if you provide a written guide to help others understand your creation.

Self-published book. You can combine several of the above methods in the form of a self-published book. For example, you can combine text and photographs and even include a CD. Self-publishing allows you to publish a single copy or as many copies of your book as you wish to print. Creating and publishing a book is not a simple task. You need to do your homework, understand what is involved in self-publishing, and decide on the level of professionalism you want to achieve.

Who Can Help You Tell Your Story

It's a lot more fun and easier if you have someone help you with telling your story, particularly if your chronic illness limits your mobility or energy. Here are some resources you can tap to find someone to assist you with your storytelling efforts.

Friend or family member. If you are serious about telling your life story and committed to getting it done, you should be able find a friend or family member to assist you. First, however, you need to get organized by deciding what you want to tell and selecting a storytelling method. Then when you ask someone to help you, you will be able to give that person a description of your vision for your story.

High school or college student. Students with an interest in history are also a good source of assistance. Working with you on creating your life story will give the student practical experience in creating a personal history. If you choose to use a more technical method of storytelling such as a video recording or a self-published book, a student will be a very helpful assistant. Their available time may be limited and you need to be organized.

StoryCorps. If you live near a StoryCorps recording facility in New York, San Francisco, or Atlanta, it can be an excellent resource for telling your story.

Local historian. A historian, especially someone who lives in your community, can be an invaluable resource to help you with your project. A historian is a storyteller by definition and can help you develop the way in which your story is told. There is no right or wrong way to tell your story but an experienced storyteller can help you explore alternative styles to find the one that best meets your personality and story.

Ways to Share Your Story

Once you have created your life story in one of the formats described previously, you are ready for the fun part of storytelling—sharing your story with the many different groups of people who will be interested in it. Here are a few ideas to get you started.

Support groups associated with your chronic illness. The essence of support is the sharing of ideas, solutions to problems unique to this illness, and giving encouragement to others in the same situation. Your life story will contain each aspect of support for similarly affected people. They will receive your story with interest and enthusiasm. The ideal way to present your story is in person.

Local media. Newspapers, magazines, radio, and television depend on a continuous stream of human-interest stories to attract their audience. At least one of them may be interested in your story. Some homework on your part (for example, has a story like yours appeared before in this medium?) will help you narrow the list of potentially interested media.

The Internet. The Internet has revolutionized how people throughout the world communicate with each other. It provides you with the means for sharing your story with anyone, anywhere on planet Earth, as long as both of you have access to some type of electronic device such as a computer, a smart phone, or a tablet device like the Apple iPad.

The Internet is a vast collection of private, public, and governmental computer networks throughout the world that can communicate with each other through e-mail, websites, and social media like Facebook and Twitter. Web pages present information in many different forms, including text, video, and images. You can use all of these electronic tools to share your story, and even build your own personal website.

Family, friends, and your healthcare team. You might invite members of your support team to a special presentation of your life story. Ask your caregiver what venue is available for a presentation.

Schools and other organizations. The term "school" can be taken in its broadest sense. Anywhere people learn about how other people manage health problems are places that may be interested in your life story, such as hospitals and clinics. Your local library, senior centers, and social organizations may have story-sharing sessions. If you look around your community, you may be pleasantly surprised by how many opportunities exist for telling your life story.

How to Organize Your Story

Below is a worksheet that will help you make a plan for your story. You may find the journalist's Five Ws method useful for organizing your story. Newspaper reporters commonly use this method to make sure that they have all the important and basic information that the reader will want to know. They use these five words to guide them in collecting information to include in the story: Who, What, When, Where, and Why.

- Who is the focus of the story?
- What do you want to say about them?
- When did the story happen?
- Where did the story take place?
- Why did it happen?

Once you've covered these five basic points, you can expand your story out from there and add as much additional information and descriptive detail as you can to help your audience get a full picture of what occurred.

WORKSHEET FOR CREATING YOUR LIFE STORY

Before you fill out this worksheet, sit quietly, close your eyes, and imagine the type of story you want to create, what you want to tell people about your life, and how you want to do it. That will help you visualize the steps and resources that you will need to carry out your project.

STEP 1. WHAT DO YOU WANT PEOPLE TO KNOW ABOUT YOU?

Think about the important events of your life, what they mean, what would be of interest to other people, and the lessons you want people to take away from your story.

STEP 2. CHOOSE THE TOPICS YOU WANT TO INCLUDE IN YOUR STORY THAT WILL CONVEY WHAT YOU WANT PEOPLE TO KNOW ABOUT YOU.

Make a list of every topic that comes to mind. Put the list away for a few days, and then come back to it and narrow it down to the topics that are most important to you. Don't overdo it—make sure you can handle the number of topics comfortably.

1. _____

2. _____

3. _____

4. _____

5. _____

STEP 3. DECIDE THE MEDIUM YOU WANT TO USE TO TELL YOUR STORY.

___ Oral presentation in person

___ Tape recording

___ Video recording

___ Written

___ Photographs with captions

___ Photographs with written stories

___ Paintings

___ Drawings

___ Music

___ Self-published book

___ Other:

STEP 4. LIST THE TOOLS YOU WILL NEED TO CREATE YOUR STORY.

Examples: computer, camera, tape recorder, CDs, etc.

1. _____

2. _____

3. _____

4. _____

5. _____

STEP 5. LIST THE PEOPLE YOU WILL ASK FOR HELP AND HOW EACH PERSON WILL HELP YOU.

1. _____

2. _____

3. _____

4. _____

5. _____

STEP 6. MAKE AN OUTLINE OF THE MAIN POINTS YOU WANT TO PRESENT. PUT THEM IN ORDER. LIST THE DETAILS UNDER EACH POINT.

Example: <u>Growing Up on a Farm in Maine in the 1930s</u>

My grandparents' farm
    Location
    The land
    Buildings: house, barn, out buildings
    Animals
    Crops

Our daily life
    Schedule for milking
    Seasonal chores: planting; harvest

Hardships
    No electricity
    Got water from a pump
    Long days of physical labor

Working outside in all weather
Winter

Why I loved the farm
    Strong family connections
    Freedom
    Being outdoors
    Working with nature
    Beautiful setting

STEP 7. CREATE YOUR STORY.

STEP 8. GET FEEDBACK ON YOUR STORY AND REVISE IT AS NECESSARY.

Ask someone whose opinion you respect and who will be honest with you about suggesting changes to review what you've created. If your story is in written form, you might seek input from an editor. You will find that writing is more fun when you have a collaborator with whom you can share your ideas and writing.

STEP 9. PRESENT YOUR STORY IN YOUR CHOSEN FORMAT AND VENUE.

Part 4

FREE YOUR SPIRIT

CHAPTER 9

Your Spiritual Journey

Your time is limited, so don't waste it living someone else's life. Don't be trapped by dogma — which is living with the results of other people's thinking. Don't let the noise of others' opinions drown out your own inner voice. And most important, have the courage to follow your heart and intuition.

> — Steve Jobs, cofounder of Apple,
> Stanford University commencement address,
> June 14, 2005, one year after being diagnosed
> with pancreatic cancer

Alex's New Spiritual Outlook

PRIOR TO HIS CANCER DIAGNOSIS, Alex had been a very active member of his church. His pastor considered him one of the most dependable members because Alex invariably said yes to whatever was asked of him. He regularly visited sick church members, and his faith was so strong that the pastor occasionally asked him to preach at a Sunday service.

After his diagnosis, Alex became less and less active at church and eventually stopped attending. It was at this time that a mutual friend introduced him to me with the idea that I would be Alex's spiritual counselor during his period of treatment. Alex was rather dubious but said he was willing to give it a try. Thus began our twice-a-month meetings as he endured many weeks of radiation and chemotherapy treatments.

After meeting with Alex, I began to realize that he was not one but two persons. I called his two personalities Mr. Inside and Mr. Outside. Whenever I spoke to him about his cancer diagnosis and treatment, he was calm (as calm as a cancer patient can be). He had done a lot of homework to understand his cancer. He told me he understood what the doctors were telling him about his treatment options and was living a lifestyle to maximize his chances of survival. That was Mr. Outside.

Mr. Inside had a fiery stream of seething emotions coursing through his veins. He was angry, fearful, grieving, and highly stressed.

Alex was very angry with God. He had been a good and faithful Christian all his life. He was committed to his church, a good husband and father, and involved in several community organizations. He didn't smoke or drink alcohol, exercised regularly, and ate moderately. Why had God done this to Alex? And why didn't God answer his prayers to cure the cancer?

Alex was very afraid of dying. He said he believed in God and the resurrection of Jesus, but that wasn't enough to overcome his intense fear of death. He wasn't able to tell me exactly what it was that he feared. He said things like, "I can't imagine everything just ending." "I've always been afraid." "If God gave me life, why is he taking it away?" "Life is so useless to end in death."

Alex was grieving the loss of the good life he enjoyed with his family before the diagnosis. In a few years, his last child would graduate from college. Then he and his wife would be empty nesters and they could retire and enjoy the happy life they had planned and saved for. Now all that planning and work had been for nothing.

As Alex's spiritual counselor, my role was to assist, not to direct him. In our discussions, he recognized how his emotions were draining the energy he wanted and needed to fight his illness. We discussed several options for venting and reducing his anger, fear, and grief. He decided to write a diary of his treatments, experiences, and feelings. After several weeks, he said the diary was giving him a way of expressing himself and that he was feeling better. I suggested he share his diary entrees with friends and family members on the Internet and ask them for their comments. By allowing others to participate in his experiences, he created his own support group.

I seemed to strike a raw nerve when I suggested that Alex write about the things that were most important to him before his cancer diagnosis. His initial reaction was a shrug of the shoulders, a tightening of the lips, and silence. Eventually he said he would think about it. I brought up the topic again a few meetings later to see if he would at least discuss the idea with me. To my surprise, he smiled and said, "I bet you thought I'd rejected your idea. I've written something for you to read." He handed me several sheets of typing.

Alex wrote about his experiences as a high school history teacher and the joy and pride he experienced in helping students to learn from the lessons of history. His essay opened the door to a discussion of what could be the purpose and meaning of his life postdiagnosis. Several meetings later, he told me that he was going to write and self-publish a book to help other cancer patients deal with the physical and mental pain and suffering that follows a cancer diagnosis.

Alex has completed his treatments and his cancer is in remission. He is again a practicing member of his church. He's not the full-of-enthusiasm, go-to guy anymore. He doesn't have the energy or desire to return to that role. He has become quiet, more reflective and spiritual. He's the one that people seek out when they're having a tough problem and need someone trustworthy to help them.

I asked Alex why he came back to church and if he was still mad at God. I think you will find his answer helpful if you are trying to increase your sense of spirituality. He said, "Before my diagnosis, I put God in the same category as Santa Claus. I thought that if I was a good Christian and asked God to rid me of my cancer, he would reward my good behavior and do as I asked. That, of course, didn't happen. Now I see God challenging me to use the gifts I've received from him. I have to take personal responsibility for dealing with the suffering and pain of my disease and at the same time find a purpose and meaning for my life, however long it is. Instead of being angry, I'm grateful for the people God sends to help me. I was a teacher before the diagnosis and now that I've returned to work I'm still a teacher. But my most important teaching responsibility is to help other cancer patients deal with their illness. That's the purpose of my book."

Alex's story shows that many personal crises offer the possibility of deep personal transformation, especially on the spiritual level. Alex used his cancer diagnosis to come to a new, more helpful understanding of his purpose in the world and of his relationship with God. Instead of closing down as he feared, his life expanded after his diagnosis into new areas that increased his sense of purpose and meaning. It was his new spiritual outlook that made that possible.

Spirituality and Chronic Illness

You didn't choose to have a chronic illness. I've never met a patient who said to me, "I really wanted to have diabetes," or "I enjoy having a chronic illness." There are some aspects of illness that are beyond your control, such as genetic causes. However, the main message of this book has been that <u>you can take control of how you respond to your illness</u>.

We have explored some of the ineffective and even harmful ways that people respond to their diagnosis of a chronic illness, such as denial and anger. I have introduced you to some powerful positive ways of dealing with your illness: dropping your excess emotional baggage, healthy grieving, reinventing yourself, strengthening your bonds with others, and positive thinking. By now you are most likely accustomed to the idea that illness brings change and that change is part and parcel of what it means to be human. You have come to understand that transformation is a positive thing, no matter how difficult it is.

I have saved for last the most powerful tool you can apply to coping with your illness and using it for transformation inside and out: your personal spirituality. In this chapter I will help you come to a simple understanding of what spirituality is and how you can use it for your well-being. If you are not a religious person or are even opposed to religion, <u>do not short-change yourself by skipping this chapter</u>. Religion and spirituality can be two different things. Don't deny yourself the tremendous benefits of a private spirituality.

A spiritual response to your illness takes into account your life goals, your values, and your present situation and utilizes all of your resources, especially your human spirit, to move you toward achieving your goals. In the end, whether you attain your goal is less important than the efforts you made attempting to reach it. In other words, "You ran the good race."

The Human Spirit

The spiritual response is your best response to your chronic illness because it will sustain you through the difficult moments, focus your efforts, motivate you to do your best whatever the circumstances, and give you the satisfaction of enjoying those aspects of life that are most important to you. All this is possible when you draw upon your human spirit.

The human spirit is an unlimited source of personal energy. Everyone is born with this tremendous resource. It allows you to focus mental and physical forces and energies on your goals. It keeps you going when you feel emotionally defeated and your conscious willpower is running low. In ordinary times and conditions, few individuals use the full potential of their human spirit, because they are unaware of just how deep their well of spiritual energy is, and they don't know how to tap into it.

Facing major adversity, as in chronic illness — particularly when confronted with their mortality — makes people search for a new reserve of strength and energy. This is the opportune time to become acquainted with your human spirit and all that it is capable of.

What Is Spirituality?

"Spirituality" is a word that can stir up strong emotions in some people who believe that only they have the correct or true understanding of what spirituality is, or in those who confuse spirituality with religion. In this book you will find no claims about the one and only spiritual truth. My goal is to help you define and live a spirituality that best fits your needs as you deal each day with your chronic illness. You may find that you share certain spiritual beliefs and practices with others. That's well and good, because there is strength in community, but community is not essential for an effective spiritual practice. It is most important that you "own" your spirituality and use it to guide you in whatever you do — today, tomorrow, and each day of your life.

Simply stated, spirituality is *a way of thinking and living* that uses the positive aspects of human thinking, feelings, and behavior to achieve meaning and purpose in life.

Spirituality is central to most religions, including Christianity, Islam, Judaism, Hinduism, and Buddhism. Each religion defines spirituality uniquely according to the teachings of that religion. In doing so, the religion provides guidelines for achieving spirituality.

But spirituality certainly can exist independently of religion! In that case, the individual takes responsibility for personally defining spirituality and proceeding along an individual path to achieving it.

A spiritual outlook and a spiritual life require certain qualities of mind, including commitment, acceptance, reflection, and gratitude.

Commitment is an essential ingredient for creating a meaningful life, especially if you are facing a multitude of personal challenges associated with your illness. I said above that spirituality is a way of living. A spiritual life is a committed life, a life that is lived according to specific values and goals that you identify for yourself.

You may say that you are too busy or have so many problems to contend with that you don't have time to think about the meaning of your life, let alone make a commitment to something that may never be achieved. Or you may say, "I want to keep my options open" to justify not choosing a direction and goal for your life. Commitment, in your mind, may be associated with risk: the possibility of making a mistake with something so important as your life.

But in fact the opposite is true. Making a commitment to define the meaning of the life that you seek has several advantages that will actually improve the quality of your life as events, activities, and demands swirl about in your mind. Choosing a course of action will:

- Simplify your life
- Reduce your stress level
- Rid your mind of doubts
- Give you tremendous strength by drawing on your human spirit
- Focus your energy
- Give you reasons for living life to its fullest

Commitment is highly personal and can be expressed in as many different ways as there are people. For some, commitment comes through their work. For others, their commitment is found in artistic expressions like musical performance, painting, sculpture, writing, poetry, or dance. For others, commitment may take the form of a hobby or involvement in a social cause. And we all show our commitment to specific values in our relationships with our loved ones and other people. Regardless of what form commitment takes, the benefits of a committed life are substantial. Making the most of this one life you have been given is a highly spiritual act.

Acceptance of yourself and others is the foundation of spiritual behavior—and it may be one of the greatest hurdles for all of us. When we see someone behaving in a way that is distinctly different from the way we ourselves behave, our mind tends to jump immediately into judgment mode. Making a judgment about someone implies that your personal values and choices are better than others', and that not sharing your values and choices diminishes another person's worth. That's a very harmful assumption because judgment blocks communication. It prevents learning, promotes ignorance, enflames negative emotions and wastes precious energy that you need for other more important uses. It also separates you from others instead of promoting connections among people.

Acceptance, on the other hand, acknowledges that things and people are the way they are and encourages you to explore the question, "Why is it so?" Acceptance doesn't mean that you agree with another person's way of being, but rather that you are open to learning and understanding. Judgment can be inflammatory and result in a hardening of your perceptions as well as a hardening of your arteries. Acceptance can be calming and result in greater awareness and understanding of how others may see the same world differently than you do.

Acceptance of yourself and your life as it is at this very moment is as important as acceptance of others. It is all too easy to become depressed over what you have lost because of your illness, what life might have been without this disease. Acknowledging your current situation—your strengths, resources, and weaknesses—will change your view from looking back at the past to looking forward to the future and what you can achieve in your life.

Reflection means stopping often to ask yourself where you are and what direction you are headed in. Are you still pursuing the life you dreamed of as a young person? Does your life reflect your values and what is important to you? Are you living a committed life? Reflection means taking responsibility for moving yourself along on your spiritual journey. You're in charge of your spirituality. If you're making good progress, that's great. If you find yourself wandering away from your goals, you need to correct your course to realign yourself with your values and your life's mission.

Gratitude is a life-transforming spiritual attitude. It is a gift that you give to yourself that enhances the quality of your life. Expressing appreciation for what others do for you is also your gift to them. People enjoy receiving gifts and you feel good in giving them.

Chronic illness involves an army of caretakers and healthcare providers to support a patient's complex needs. In trying to deal with all these problems, it is easy to become self-centered and come to expect people to take care of you. It's important that you acknowledge their efforts on your behalf in a heartfelt way. When you take an interest in those who care for you, you are acknowledging that they are individuals who have their own lives, needs, and concerns. Expressing your gratitude in words or actions enhances their lives and reminds you that you are always part of a loop of giving and receiving that has its roots in the spiritual concept of caring for one another.

What Spirituality Can Do for You

There are very practical reasons for adopting a spiritual mindset and spiritual behaviors. The most important reason is the effect spirituality has on your view of life, beginning with enhancing your optimism. Humans are naturally optimistic. Chronic illness, however, can smother optimism with a blanket of darkness, sadness, and depression. Spirituality allows optimism to overcome negative emotions and helps you see that your future can be brighter than you once thought. Optimism gives you strength to move ahead. Recent scientific studies have found that optimistic people can live healthier and longer lives.

Spirituality can bring about a greater willingness to forgive yourself and others. An inability to forgive is one if the biggest pieces of excess emotional baggage that people carry around. As we've discussed before, grudges are associated with anger and stress. Letting go of long-held hard feelings and perceptions can be very hard for some people, but it is essential to achieving the inner peace associated with spirituality. Like charity, forgiveness begins at home — that is, with yourself. Until you have forgiven yourself for past transgressions, it is doubtful that you can truly forgive others. You have to love and accept yourself in order to love and accept others.

Spirituality can help you confront and calm your fears. Uppermost of all fears, especially for chronically ill patients, is the fear of death. In the United States, death has become a taboo social topic. We don't mention the words "death" or "dying" anymore. We use euphemisms such as "passing" and "departed." It's not a topic of common discussion among family members and friends because death is not as frequently experienced in our society as it was only a century ago. Improvements in medicine have brought about dramatic changes in longevity. This has created an expectation among Americans that science can extend life indefinitely. Death has come to be considered an unfortunate intrusion rather than a natural event.

The spiritual person is more likely to develop a personal philosophy regarding death that brings a sense of calm and peace in the final stage of life. Your personal philosophy might include an understanding of the meaning of your life and how it unfolds over time, from birth to death, and perhaps an idea of what awaits you after death.

An unwillingness to acknowledge and address one's mortality creates a fear of death. By the time a patient arrives at a hospice, it is usually too late for pastoral counseling to deal with this intense emotion. This was true of Jim. His brother, Joe, told me after the funeral that Jim's last words were, "This is a terrible way to die." It was true that Joe died in physical and emotional pain. He admitted to me that he had an intense fear of death. He never moved beyond that fear and it dominated the last eighteen months of his life, beginning with his denial of his cancer. In chapter one we saw, through the stories of Sharon and of Randy Pausch, that how you think about death can dramatically alter your quality of life in your final weeks and months.

This is true for everyone, no matter how we die. We all want comfort and peace in the last phase of our life. Understanding the meaning and purpose of death will help you be open to receiving that comfort. The meaning and purpose of death is an important question that you need to answer for yourself by thinking deeply about your values, beliefs, and experiences. Don't leave that discussion with yourself for the last moment.

Sister Ann waged a battle against the cancer in her body for about the same length of time as Jim did. She too had an endless stream of visitors, but her demeanor, in contrast, was uplifted and joyful. Her goal in life was to live to be ninety years old. I visited her weekly in her final months. One day, she told me, "God is my pal and I'll be seeing my pal soon." During her stay in the hospice, the staff was unable to transport her to the chapel for daily Mass. On her ninetieth birthday, I conducted a service in her room for her and members of her community. We sang her favorite hymns and she participated by tapping her toe in rhythm with our singing. A few days later, she died calmly and peacefully.

Sister Ann's specific beliefs about God and the afterlife were essential elements of a spiritual philosophy that sustained her in life, kept her moving toward her goal of living a long and good life, and filled her with peace and even joy as she approached her death without fear. You can use your spirituality to control your fears, including the fear of death, and free yourself to do what is most meaningful for you.

How Spirituality Can Help You Deal with Chronic Illness

I want to make a very important distinction between spirituality and "faith healing." You should not adopt spiritual behavior with an expectation that doing so will change the course of your illness. That is something you and your team of healthcare providers are working on.

Having said that, there is a scientific reason why spirituality and faith can benefit your health. In the brain the hypothalamus and pituitary gland are responsible for managing the release of hormones into the blood stream, hormones that regulate every aspect of the body's activities and vitality. Spirituality heals the mind, which, in turn, causes the release of hormones that benefit your physical condition. That may even reduce your level of pain.

Spiritual people tend to be optimistic people. Optimism buoys up the spirit and brightens your outlook on life. One study of comparable middle-aged cancer patients found that optimistic patients outlived pessimistic patients.

A spiritual mindset also lowers your stress level by eliminating unnecessary and burdensome negative emotions. Continuous high levels of stress have been shown to adversely affect the immune system — the body's main line of defense against disease. Reducing your stress level increases your resistance to disease and aids your body in fighting your illness.

Perhaps the greatest health benefit spirituality can offer is an increased openness to change. The ever-constant companion of chronic illness is change, some anticipated and much that seem to come out of nowhere. As you attempt to maintain some sense of normalcy, you may experience an increasing resistance to change, including changes in treatment. Sometimes you may be tempted to say, "Just leave me alone. I don't want to make any more changes." A spiritual outlook can help you accept and adapt to necessary changes.

Regardless of your specific religious beliefs, your spirituality can make you feel connected to the world outside yourself —

to people, to the natural world, to whatever your understanding of a creator is. Having those connections, you feel less alone. You sense that you don't have to rely only on your own limited resources; you can draw from the strength of those connections. Your faith in your connectedness can get you through the hardest challenges in dealing with your illness and give you the courage to carry on and squeeze as much living as you can out of the remainder of your existence.

You, God, and Chronic Illness

Life with a chronic illness raises fundamental questions about life that may not have concerned you before your diagnosis:

- Does being chronically ill serve any purpose?
- Can there be meaning in a life of chronic illness?
- How do I avoid becoming a burden on others?
- What social value does a chronically ill person have?

"These are really tough questions. How do I begin to answer them?" you ask. The starting point is yet another question: What is your relationship to God? That is, what do you believe?

A major study of American religious beliefs by the Pew Forum found that nearly eight out of ten Americans believe in God. Approximately two out of ten Americans do not believe in God. (A small percent of the respondents indicated a religious affiliation that was not God centered.)

For some people, answering these questions about their relationship to God will not be difficult. For others, it will require a dose of courage because it means confronting your own existence and mortality. The purpose of exploring your relationship to God and your other beliefs, whether religious or not, is to create a philosophical compass to guide you in making the tough decisions that are a part of living with chronic illness. Answering these questions for yourself can lead to spiritual insights that lift you above and beyond the constraints of your illness.

Achieving a Spiritual State of Mind

Whether you are just thinking about becoming more spiritual or are already on your journey, it will be welcome news to know that everyone has the potential to develop the essential personal attributes for spirituality. Most importantly, you need to be committed to reflection and open to learning new ideas that will deepen your understanding of yourself and your place in the world.

There are many sources of spiritual understanding. They can be generally classified as internal and external: understanding that you come to through private reflection, and knowledge and insights that you learn from other sources, including secular and religious books, the philosophy of your established religion if you have one, discussion with others, and so on.

Private reflection can take the form of meditation, prayer, writing, or just plain thinking. In your reflective moments, take the time first to find out what spiritual questions are most important for you. Common spiritual questions pertain to our origin, our purpose in this life, the existence and role of a creator, the soul, why life seems to be so fraught with difficulty, exactly how we should live our lives, and what happens when we die.

Finding answers to those questions is the work of a lifetime, but it will be helpful if you can begin by stating what understanding you are seeking, even if your answers to some of the above questions is, "I just don't know."

Although I have emphasized that spirituality is highly personal, and I am intentionally avoiding sharing my own beliefs with you because I want you to make your own spiritual discoveries, it is nonetheless true that humans have been thinking about spiritual questions for thousands of years and you can benefit from the vast existing knowledge and understanding of spirituality written down and taught over the centuries. Amazon.com currently lists more than 160,000 books on religion and spirituality!

You will be wise to choose your sources of external spiritual learning carefully, including the books you read, lectures you attend, and so on. Listen and read with good judgment. Keep an open mind, but listen to your intuition and apply your reason.

You may decide at some point that you are in need of personal spiritual guidance, especially if you are blocked by a thorny question or predicament. This can be found from leaders of a religious organization (church, synagogue, mosque, or other place of worship) or other spiritual movement. Some spiritual counselors have specific training in assisting individual spiritual development. Be sure to check the counselor's credentials and work only with someone that you truly trust. Choose teachers who have spiritual qualities that you want to acquire and who can serve as a role model. Look for the true message and motives beneath a teacher's external presentation — charisma is no indication of spiritual wisdom. What has been that person's own spiritual journey? What challenges has the person had to overcome that have led to special wisdom? Is this person living a values-based life that you can identify with? Does the spiritual teacher support your personal learning journey?

Your Personal Spiritual Values

Your specific spiritual questions and your (clear or tentative) answers will lead to a system of personal beliefs. Knowing what you believe (at least at this point in time) will lead you logically to a set of values that are compatible with your beliefs and that guide how you live your life. For example, if you believe that we were put on this earth to help one another, then compassion will be high on your list of values, and compassion will guide your decision making and your actions.

Personal values are at the heart of how you conduct your life: your goals, your choice of occupation, your relationships, how you solve problems, how you spend your money, how you spend your leisure time, and much more. I have defined spirituality as a *positive* way of thinking and living to achieve meaning and purpose in life. That definition points to specific spiritual values, such as kindness, compassion, generosity, respect for others, caring for the planet and for all living things. Those values pertain to how you relate to the world. Other values are about your character and personal standards: courage, responsibility, persistence, never giving up even in the face of defeat, making the most of the time you've been given in this life, expanding your mind, how you care for yourself, and so on. The more you are aware of your personal values, the better you will be able to design your life around those values.

Personal values evolve over your lifetime, but they are still there even in a time of challenge and illness. For example, if you value doing as much as you can with your life, that value will continue to push you forward even as your circumstances change. You will simply find new ways to express your values.

Spirituality Is Meant to Be Lived

By now you understand that spirituality is much more than attendance at a place of worship, or knowing the dogma of a specific religion. Spirituality is meant to pervade every aspect of your life on a daily basis. It asks one simple question of you: How are you going to live out this life, today and every day? A serious illness can make you aware of the importance of that question in ways that you never realized before. Suddenly you realize how precious each day is, and you ask how you can make the most of it. You ask what is most important for you now, in these changed circumstances. Your growing spiritual sense calls for deeper answers than you may have given in the past.

Many of the stories in this book have illustrated that chronically ill people who come to a new understanding of what is important in life often choose to give as much as they can to other people. They stop being preoccupied with all the details of their own life and focus instead on making things easier for others. They choose to live on the higher spiritual plane of giving and to leave that as their legacy.

We all have the potential for spiritual greatness. Spiritual greatness is not the same as being recognized for your accomplishments on the world stage. Spiritual greatness means making the most of whatever you have been endowed with, constantly growing in your understanding, and giving as much as you can to the world. You can achieve spiritual greatness by continually reflecting on how you are living and putting your values into practice every day, in every way you can find. Hold yourself to a high standard, so that everything you say and do is consistent with your spiritual values. Put your beliefs and values into action at every opportunity.

Your Spiritual Journey Is Never Finished

In chapter 3 you learned that Life Is Change. We all inherit a set of beliefs and values from our family and our culture. A spiritual outlook calls us to examine our inherited beliefs and values and make sure they are aligned with who we are as individuals, in this place and time, and that they are helping us live better lives. Values and beliefs are not static;

they become deeper and more complex as we mature. Fortunately, we are endowed with intelligent minds to engage in that continual process of examination. On-going reflection and being open to new understanding are at the core of a truly spiritual practice and a spiritual life.

CHAPTER 10

Ten Powerful Insights for Moving Beyond a Chronic Illness and Living Life to the Fullest

1. *There is life beyond your chronic illness and it is yours to live.* Wanting to live beyond your illness is what prompted you to pick up this book. The question is, what are you going to do with this *new* life? You can respond positively to your illness and work your way to a new perspective, or you can become mired in negative emotions and surrender to them. As Mary Oliver expresses it in her poem, "The Summer Day," "Tell me, what is it you plan to do with your one wild and precious life?"

2. *"Carpe diem"—Seize the day.* Please make a large sign with this motto and put it where you will see it every morning. Today is the only day you have. Yesterday is no more. Tomorrow may or may not arrive. Hold on to today with all your strength. Make it a day worth remembering by

focusing on what is most important to you. Do as much as you can of whatever is meaningful and fulfilling for you. If it is also meaningful and fulfilling to others, so much the better. At the end of the day, have the satisfaction of saying, "This was truly a good day. A day worth living."

3. *Others will help—but only if you reach out to them.* You are not alone in the battle to fight your illness. There is an army of healthcare providers, counselors, advocates, caregivers, family, and friends who are willing to help you. But you first have to acknowledge their presence, ask for their assistance, and work with them.

4. *Control fear or it will control you.* Fear is a natural response to learning that you have a serious illness. If allowed to become an overwhelming negative emotion, it will paralyze you and lead to bad mental and physical health decisions. Instead, confront your fear. Describe what you are afraid of and it will shrink to manageable proportions. Use the techniques described in this book to manage negative emotions. Most importantly, don't be afraid of asking for help to conquer your fear. Don't surrender to fear. Be brave, gather your forces, and do battle.

5. *The antidote to loneliness is found in the heart of a friend, not in a bottle or pill.* The loneliness of chronic illness can be very painful. You can't drown loneliness in alcohol or other abuses; that only makes things worst. Reach out to people in as many ways as you can think of. Make new friends to make up for those who no longer call you. Volunteering, sup-

port groups, and activity groups are your best sources for meeting new people.

6. *Take responsibility for your actions and improve your health.* You are responsible for doing all you can to take care of yourself mentally and physically. How you care for yourself determines what your healthcare team can do to assist you. If you act responsibly, there is a great deal they can do for you.

7. *Cast off negative emotions and enjoy a calm mind and peaceful heart.* Negative emotions divert critical energy from your thinking brain to your emotional brain. The more negative emotions you carry, the less rational you become. Get rid of your negative emotions and the resulting calm and peace will give you a clearer and better vision of the present and your future.

8. *Be resilient.* Visualize yourself as the full-of-energy bunny in the TV commercials that keeps going and going. You can achieve a new perspective and live a full life. But you have to be able to get up and get going again when something trips you up. In chronic illness, there are endless obstructions that can stop you from moving ahead. Your determination to go around them and keep moving is your badge of courage.

9. *Do something enjoyable every day.* What makes you smile, laugh, relax, and feel good? What takes you out of an illness mood and makes you happy? What's your favorite happy activity—listening to music, going for a walk, reading

a book, chatting with a friend, watching a good movie? Whatever it is, do something every day that makes you happy. It will make you glad to be alive.

10. *Spirituality will give you wings to fly over your illness*. The trials and tribulations of a chronic illness can trap you in a mental cocoon of negativity, a virtual prison. You have the greatest source of energy on earth at your disposal: your human spirit. Use it to break free of your illness mindset and let your spirituality raise you to a height where you can see what opportunities await you. This is possible and achievable. Believe and it will happen.

Afterword

I hope that you have found in this book many new ways of thinking about not only your chronic illness, but your life as a whole, for your illness is but one element of all you are as a person and of the life you have lived so far and the life yet to come. I would like to leave you with this simple poem often attributed to Ralph Waldo Emerson, which expresses in just a few words how you will know when you have expanded your vision beyond your chronic illness. I wish you well from this point forward. May you know success as this poem paints it.

SUCCESS

To laugh often and much;

To win the respect of intelligent people and the affection of children;

To earn the appreciation of honest critics and endure the betrayal of false friends;

To appreciate beauty,

To find the best in others,

To leave the world a bit better, whether by a healthy child, a garden patch or a redeemed social condition;

To know even one life has breathed easier because you have lived.

This is to have succeeded.

Endnotes

1 Jeffrey Zaslow, "A Beloved Professor Delivers the Lecture of a Lifetime," *Wall Street Journal*, September 20, 2007.

2 Thomas Cathcart and Daniel Klein, *Heidegger and a Hippo Walk Through Those Pearly Gates* (New York: Penguin Books, 2009), p. 34.

3 *Flourish: A Visionary New Understanding of Happiness and Well-Being* (New York: Free Press, 2011).

4 Martin E. P. Seligman and Mihaly Csikszentmihalyi, "Introduction to Positive Psychology," *American Psychologist* 55, no. 1 (Jan. 2000): 5–14.

5 Jessica Colman, *Optimal Functioning: A Positive Psychology Handbook* (Kindle edition, Jan. 2011).

6 Ein-shei Chen, "An Example of Home Care: The Case of Chen Ein-Shei" (presentation, International Symposium on Research on Home Care of Patients with ALS in East Asia, Ritsumeikan University, Kyoto, Japan, February 21, 2009).

7 Ibid.

8 Television program on ALS patients aired in Taiwan on 10/15/11, http://www.youtube.com/watch?v=iRZDr2doPow&feature=related accessed 2/1/12

9 Stephen Hawking, "Disability Advice," www.hawking.org.uk/index.php/disability

[10] John Boslough, *Stephen Hawking's Universe: An Introduction to the Most Remarkable Scientist of Our Time* (New York: Quill, 1985).

[11] Retrieved from http://www.youtube.com/watch?v=PrJVbCzJH6c

[12] *New York Times*, August 25, 2008. Retrieved from http://www.nytimes.com/2008/08/26/us/politics/26text-kennedy.html

[13] Thomas K. Houston et al., "Culturally Appropriate Storytelling to Improve Blood Pressure: A Randomized Trial." *Annals of Internal Medicine*, vol. 154, no. 2 (January 18, 2011): 78–95.

362.19   Cheu, Richard
C526   Living well with
          chronic illness

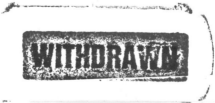

CPSIA information can be obtained at www.ICGtesti
Printed in the USA
LVOW10s1536140813

347874LV00002B/258/P